中国农业科学院智库报告

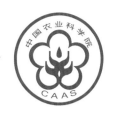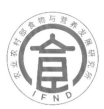

2022年中国食物与营养发展报告

China Food and Nutrition Development Report 2022

农业农村部食物与营养发展研究所　编著

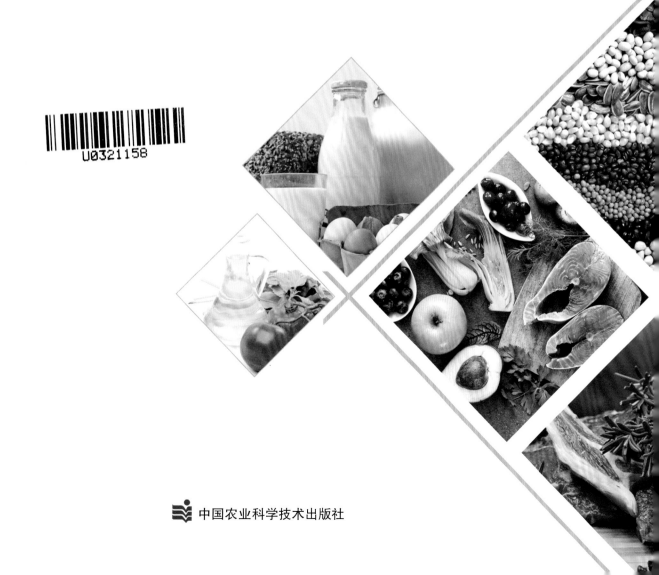

中国农业科学技术出版社

图书在版编目（CIP）数据

2022 年中国食物与营养发展报告 / 农业农村部食物与营养发展研究所编著 . -- 北京：中国农业科学技术出版社，2023.6

ISBN 978-7-5116-6298-9

Ⅰ. ① 2⋯　　Ⅱ. ①农⋯　　Ⅲ. ①食品营养—发展—研究—中国—2022　　Ⅳ. ① R151.3

中国国家版本馆 CIP 数据核字（2023）第 097850 号

责任编辑　史咏竹
责任校对　马广洋
责任印制　姜义伟　王思文

出 版 者　中国农业科学技术出版社
　　　　　北京市中关村南大街 12 号　　邮编：100081
电　　话　（010）82105169（编辑室）　　（010）82109702（发行部）
　　　　　（010）82109709（读者服务部）
网　　址　https://castp.caas.cn
经 销 者　各地新华书店
印 刷 者　北京地大彩印有限公司
开　　本　210 mm × 285 mm　1/16
印　　张　6.25
字　　数　98 千字
版　　次　2023 年 6 月第 1 版　2023 年 6 月第 1 次印刷
定　　价　56.00 元

《2022 年中国食物与营养发展报告》
编著委员会

China Food and Nutrition Development Report 2022
Editorial Board

前　言

　　改革开放 40 余年来，我国在保障国家粮食安全和居民营养健康方面取得了巨大成就，粮食产量连续 7 年保持在 1.3 万亿斤（1 斤 = 0.5 千克）以上，食物供给丰富多样，居民营养状况明显改善，全面建成小康社会。与此同时，社会经济的发展、人民日益增长的美好生活需要对食物和营养发展提出了更高更新的要求。

　　2022 年，习近平总书记在看望参加全国政协十三届五次会议的农业界、社会福利和社会保障界委员时强调，要树立大食物观。要从更好满足人民美好生活需要出发，掌握人民群众食物结构变化趋势，在确保粮食供给的同时，保障肉类、蔬菜、水果、水产品等各类食物有效供给，缺了哪样也不行。要积极推进农业供给侧结构性改革，全方位、多途径开发食物资源，开发丰富多样的食物品种，实现各类食物供求平衡，更好满足人民群众日益多元化的食物消费需求。大食物观的提出坚持了以人民为中心的发展思想，深化了以往的粮食安全观，遵循了人类发展的历史观，体现了人与自然和谐共生的自然观，彰显了人类命运共同体的视野。树立和践行大食物观，对保障我国粮食安全、提升国民营养水平、促进乡村振兴具有重要意义。

　　在国家食物与营养咨询委员会和中国农业科学院的领导和支持下，农业农村部食物与营养发展研究所围绕如何推进落实大食物观开展了系列专题研究，组织撰写了《2022 年中国食物与营养发展报告》，全面总结了改革开放以来我国食物与营养发展变化趋势，梳理研判了当前我国食物与营养领域存在的问题与挑战，最后提出了一系列保障国家食物安全、改善居民营养状况、建设健康中国的重大政策建议，以期为相关部门、食物营养相关领域从业者和关心食物与营养发展的广大读者提供借鉴和参考。报告共分三部分：第一部分为"从吃饱到吃好"；第二部分为"问题与挑战"；第三部分为"向营养健康转型"。

第一部分回顾了从吃饱到吃好的历程。自改革开放以来，我国食物生产和供给量显著增加。总体呈现三个特点。一是数量够：2021 年，粮食产量达到 6.8 亿吨，其他食物产量稳步增长，人均粮食供给量近 600 千克，食物供给充足，种类丰富。二是能量足：在营养供给方面，能量、蛋白质及脂肪供给量持续增长，特别是来源于动物性食物的营养供给呈快速增长趋势。居民人均每日能量供给量达到 3 400 千卡（1 千卡 ≈ 4.184 千焦），能够满足居民营养健康需求。三是结构尚不合理：在生产供给方面，粮食、蔬菜、水果、肉类基本自给；大豆、植物油、奶类和饲料粮进口量大幅上升。在食物消费方面，精加工谷物消费量趋于稳定，全谷物消费偏低，杂粮消费减少；肉类、蛋类、水产品消费不断增加，奶类消费仍然偏少；蔬菜、水果消费持续快速增长，为居民营养改善作出了贡献，但食用油和食糖的快速增长则可能带来健康风险。

第二部分通过分析认为，随着城乡居民收入的不断提高，人民群众对食物的消费需求日益多元化，对营养健康的关注日益迫切，但受农业发展尚未完全实现现代化、投入不足、科研力量薄弱、食育不到位等因素的影响，我国仍存在一些亟待解决的食物与营养问题。一是居民膳食不平衡，居民超重肥胖问题不断凸显，慢性病患病、发病仍呈上升趋势。主要表现为能量摄入过多导致的营养过剩和维生素A、钙、铁等营养素摄入不足导致的营养缺乏并存，油、盐、糖摄入偏高。二是过度加工导致食物营养损失较大，全产业链食物损耗浪费严重。三是居民食物营养认知转变相对滞后，合理膳食的消费理念有待强化。四是营养安全支持体系薄弱，食物资源数据匮乏，缺乏监测评价标准，食物营养品质数据库尚不完善，限制了食物资源的高质量利用、食物品种多样性的开发和居民营养改善。

第三部分围绕推进落实大食物观，提出了一系列向营养健康转型的重大政策建议。踏上新征程，我国食物与营养发展已经进入营养健康的新阶段，要以大食物观为指导，按照"转导向、调结构、树理念、强支撑"的总体思路，为保障粮食安全、推进乡村振兴和建设健康中国作出新贡献。一是加快推动营养导向型农业发展。以可持续发展为目标，以营养导向为理念，以资源禀赋为出发点，加快食物系统转型，推进营养导向型生产体系、加工体系和消费体系建设，发展营养导向型农业。二是打造第三口粮。通过加大全谷物食品开发力度，优化杂粮区域布局，推动杂粮产业提质增效，引导增加全谷物和杂粮消费，打造第三口粮，提升主食多样性，确保国家粮食安全。三是实施白肉增长计划。制定促进禽肉和水产品发展的政策，加强家禽、水产品的新品种创制和养殖关键核心技术创新，推动产业向规模化、标准化、智能化发展。多措并举，推动白肉消费和健康低碳饮食。四是积极推动食物全产业链减损节约。在从农田到餐桌的过程中多管齐下，努力减少食物损耗浪费。五是从娃娃和掌勺人开始狠抓健康饮食教育。把握好食育进校园、进家庭两个关键环节。强化主流媒体和权威机构的食育主导地位，加大主流科普团队培养。六是大力加强食物与营养科技创新。开展食物资源普查，尽快摸清家底。统筹各方力量，构建食物监测评价体系，加大食物营养品质和人体营养需求数据库建设力度。加强食物资源基础研究、技术创新和示范应用，精准挖掘不同食物资源的独特作用，充分发挥其营养健康价值。

编著者

2022 年 9 月

Preface

Over the past 40 years of reform and opening-up, China has made great achievements in ensuring national food security and residents' nutrition health. The grain production has remained above 0.65 trillion kg for 7 consecutive years. The food supply is rich and diverse, the nutritional status of residents has improved obviously, and a well-off society has been built in an all-around way. At the same time, the development of the social economy and people's growing need for a better life put forward higher and newer requirements for food and nutrition development.

In 2022, when visiting the members of the agricultural community, social welfare, and social security community who attended the 5th Session of the 13th Chinese People's Political Consultative Conference (CPPCC), General Secretary Xi Jinping emphasized that we should establish a concept of "Greater food". To better meet people's needs for a better life, we should grasp the changing trend of people's food structure, and ensure the effective supply of meat, vegetables, fruits, aquatic products, and other kinds of food while ensuring the food supply, without missing anyone. It is necessary to actively promote the structural reform of the agricultural supply side, develop food resources in all directions and many ways, develop rich and diverse food varieties, achieve the balance between supply and demand of all kinds of food, and better meet the increasingly diversified food consumption needs of the people. The concept of "Greater food" adheres to the people-centered development thinking, deepens the previous food security concept, follows the historical human development view, embodies the natural view of harmonious coexistence between man and nature, and highlights the Community of Shared Future for Mankind's vision. It is of great significance to establish and practice the concept of "Greater food" for ensuring food security in China, improving the national nutrition level, and promoting rural revitalization.

Under the leadership and support of the National Food and Nutrition Advisory Committee and the China Academy of Agricultural Sciences, the Institute of Food and Nutrition Development of the Ministry of Agriculture and Rural Affairs has conducted a series of special studies on how to promote the implementation of the concept of "Greater food", organized and written the *China Food and Nutrition Development Report 2022*. The report has comprehensively summarized the development and changing trend of food and nutrition in China since the reform and opening-up, sorted out and judged the problems and challenges existing in current food and nutrition field in China, and finally put forward a series of major policy suggestions to ensure national food safety, improve residents' nutritional status, build the "Healthy China". It aims to provide a reference for relevant departments, practitioners in food and nutrition related fields, and readers who care about the development of food and nutrition. The report is divided into three parts: the first part is "from eating-full to eating-well", the second part is "the problems and challenges"; the third part is "the transition to nutrition and health".

The first part reviews the course from eating-full to eating-well. Since the reform and opening-up, food production and supply in China have increased significantly. There are three characteristics. First, the production is sufficient. In 2021, the grain production has reached 680 million tons, and the output of other foods has increased steadily, with the per capita grain supply of 600 kg. The food supply is plentiful and varied. Second, the energy is enough. In terms of nutrition supply, the supplies of energy, protein, and fat keep increasing, especially the nutrition supply from animal food shows a rapid growth trend. The per capita daily energy supply reaches 3,400 kcal, which can meet the nutrition and health needs of residents. Third, the structure is not reasonable. In terms of production supply, grain, vegetables, fruits and meat are self-sufficient. Imports of soybeans, vegetable oils, milk and feed grains have increased substantially. In terms of food consumption, the consumption of refined grains tends to be stable, the consumption of whole grains is low, and the consumption of coarse grains is reduced. The consumption of meats, eggs and aquatic products is increasing, while the consumption of milk is still low. The consumption of vegetables and fruits continues to grow rapidly, contributing to the improvement of residents' nutrition, however, the rapid growth of edible oil and sugar consumption may bring health risks.

The analysis in the second part holds that, with the increasing income of urban and rural residents, people's demand for food is diversified, and their concern for nutrition and health is increasingly urgent. However, due to the factors such as incomplete modernization of agricultural development, insufficient investment, weak scientific research, inadequate diet education, etc., there are still some food and nutrition problems in China that need to be solved urgently. First, the diet of residents is unbalanced, the problem of overweight and obesity among residents is constantly highlighted, and the morbidity of chronic diseases is still on the rise. It is mainly characterized by both over-nutrition caused by excessive energy intake, and nutritional deficiency caused by insufficient intake of vitamin A, calcium, iron, and other micronutrients, as well as the high intake of oil, salt and sugar. Second, over-processing leads to a large loss of food nutrition. The food loss and waste in the whole industrial chain are serious. Third, the cognition of residents on food nutrition is lagging, and the consumption concept of a reasonable diet needs to be strengthened. Fourth, the nutrition and food safety support system are weak. The food resource data are scarce. The monitoring and evaluation standards are missing. The database of food nutrition quality is imperfect, which limits the high-quality utilization of food resources, the development of food variety diversity, and the improvement of residents' nutrition status.

The third part puts forward a series of major policy suggestions for the transition to nutrition and health, concerning the promotion and implementation of the "Greater food" concept. On new journey, the food and nutrition development in China has entered a new stage of nutrition and health. Guided by the concept of "Greater food", we should make new contributions to ensure food security, promote rural revitalization and build a "Healthy China" following the general idea of "changing orientation, adjusting structure, cultivating ideas, and strengthening support". First, the development of nutrition-oriented agriculture should be accelerated. With sustainable development as the goal, nutrition orientation as the concept, and resource endowment as the starting point, we will accelerate the transformation of the food system, promote the construction of a nutrition-oriented production system, processing system and consumption system, and develop nutrition-oriented agriculture. Second, the third ration can be developed. By increasing the development of cereal food, optimizing the regional layout of miscellaneous grains, promoting the quality and efficiency of the miscellaneous grain industry, guiding the increase of consumption of whole grains and miscellaneous grains, developing the third ration, enhancing the diversity of staple foods, thus ensuring national food security. Third, the white meat growth plan can be implemented. Formulating policies to promote the development of poultry meats and aquatic products, strengthening the creation of new varieties of poultry and aquatic products as well as the innovation of core technologies in breeding, promoting the scale, standardization, and intelligence of industry development. Multiple measures should be taken to promote both white meat consumption and a healthy low-carbon diet. Fourth, the reduction and saving along the whole food industry chain should be actively promoted. We should strive to reduce food loss and waste by taking multiple approaches in the process from farmland to table. Fifth, healthy diet education should be performed on children and person who cooks. We should pay attention to two key links, which are diet education in campus and family. The leading position of mainstream media and authoritative organizations in diet education should be strengthened, and the training of mainstream science popularization teams should be increased. Sixth, scientific and technological innovation in food and nutrition should be vigorously strengthened. Carrying out a general survey of food resources. All parties should coordinate their efforts to establish a food monitoring and evaluation system, and strengthen the database construction of food nutritional quality and human nutritional needs. The fundamental research, technological innovation, and demonstration application of food resources can be strengthened. The unique functions of different food resources can be accurately explored, thus maximizing their nutritional and health value.

Editors
September 2022

目　录

Contents

一

从吃饱到吃好

（一）食物产量显著增长，供给数量足够

1. 粮食产量稳定在 6.5 亿吨以上，其他食物持续增长

改革开放以来，我国食物产量稳步提升，保障了口粮供给。我国粮食的生产量呈逐年上升趋势，2021 年粮食产量达到 68 284.8 万吨，比 1980 年的 32 055.5 万吨增长 1.1 倍。菜篮子不断充实，蔬菜、水果、肉蛋奶及水产品产量快速增加。2021 年，蔬菜、水果产量分别达 77 548.8 万吨和 29 970.2 万吨，比 1980 年分别增长 14.0 倍和 43.0 倍；肉、蛋、奶及水产品产量分别为 8 990.0 万吨、3 408.8 万吨、3 682.7 万吨和 6 463.7 万吨，比 1980 年分别增长 6.5 倍、11.0 倍、31.3 倍和 13.4 倍；水果和奶类增速最快，增长 30 倍以上。油料和食糖产量持续增加。油料产量由 1980 年的 769.1 万吨增长至 2021 年的 3 586.4 万吨，增长 3.7 倍；食用植物油产量由 1980 年的 331.7 万吨增长至 2021 年的 2 855.0 万吨，增长 7.6 倍；食糖产量由 1980 年的 349.4 万吨增长至 2021 年的 1 374.5 万吨，增长近 3 倍（图 1-1）。

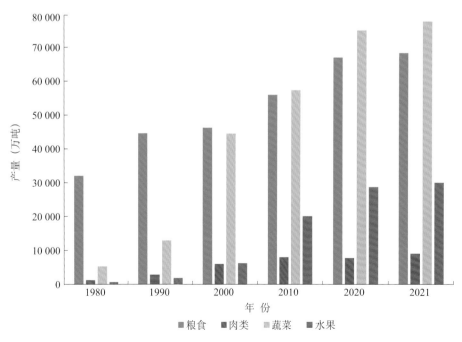

图 1-1　1980—2021 年中国主要食物产量

2. 2000 年后油料及其制品、奶类和饲料粮进口快速增长

1980—2000 年，我国粮食由净进口 1 183.7 万吨转为净出口 102.3 万吨（表 1-1）；水果、蔬菜净出口量分别增长到 56.6 万吨和 380.5 万吨，分别增长了 1.2 倍和 6.8 倍；蛋类净出口量先降后升，在 3.8 万～6.8 万吨波动；油料由净出口 11.5 万吨转为净进口 230.8 万吨；食用植物油净进口量增长到 204.4 万吨，增长了 10.2 倍；食糖净进口量下降到 157.0 万吨，下降了 76.7%；肉类净进口量达到 29.0 万吨；奶类净进口量增长到 40.1 万吨，增长了 12.8 倍；水产品净进口量则大幅增加至 459.0 万吨，增长了 167.2 倍。

2000 年以后，特别是我国加入世界贸易组织（WTO）以来，大豆、棕榈油和饲料粮进口快速增加。2021 年，粮食净进口量增加至 16 265.0 万吨，其中大豆进口量达到 1 亿吨左右；水果净出口量在 2010 年达到峰值后开始回落，2021 年首次转为净进口，当年净进口量达到 112.0 万吨；蔬菜净出口量则一路上升至 2021 年的 1 062.0 万吨，增长了 1.8 倍；油料净进口量达到 553.2 万吨；食用植物油净进口量达到 1 027.0 万吨，增长了 4.0 倍；食糖净进口量达到 621.0 万吨，增长了 3.0 倍；肉类净进口量达到 730.8 万吨，增长了 24.2 倍；奶类净进口量增至 2 195.0 万吨，增长了 5.3 倍；水产品净进口量降至 195.0 万吨，下降 57.5%。

表 1-1　1980—2021 年中国主要食物净进口量

年份	净进口量（万吨）				
	粮食	油料	食用植物油	肉类	奶类
1980	1 183.7	−11.5	18.3	−24.4	2.9
1990	798.2	−64.8	206.4	−47.1	22.8
2000	−102.3	230.8	204.4	29.0	40.1
2010	5 991.1	169.5	922.1	3.7	349.9
2020	14 205.6	570.3	966.0	789.8	1 808.0
2021	16 265.0	553.2	1 027.0	730.8	2 195.0

注：2021 年粮食净进口量数据来自《中国农业展望报告（2022—2031）》中粮食大类进出口数据；2020 年粮食净进口量数据由海关各类粮食进出口数据加总而得；其他年份粮食净进口量为联合国粮食及农业组织（FAO）食物平衡表中的谷物、薯类、杂豆和大豆四类作物加总而得。

3. 食物供给量大幅上升，数量充足，种类丰富

1980—2021 年，我国粮食供给量呈逐年上升趋势，由 33 239.2 万吨增长至 82 280.2 万吨，增长了 1.5 倍。2021 年，水果、蔬菜供给量分别达 30 082.2 万吨和 76 486.8 万吨，比 1980 年分别增长 46.0 倍和 14.5 倍。食用植物油 2021 年增长至 3 882 万吨，比 1980 年增长了约 10 倍。食糖供给量 2021 年增长至 1 995.5 万吨，比 1980 年增长近 1 倍。肉、蛋、奶及水产品 2021 年分别达到 9 720.8 万吨、3 398.8 万吨、5 877.7 万吨和 6 658.7 万吨，比 1980 年分别增长 7.2 倍、11.0 倍、49.2 倍和 14.0 倍。在供给数量大幅上升的同时，食物种类越来越丰富，多种水果、海鲜进入百姓餐盘。

粮食的人均供给量由 1980 年的 337.8 千克增加至 2021 年的 598.5 千克，接近 600 千克（表 1-2）。粮食自给率由 1980 年的 95.9% 增长至 2000 年的 100.2%，后下降至 2021 年的 85.6%，其中，大豆自给率由 1980 年的 94.8% 下降至 2021 年的 14.5%。肉类自给率略有下降，由 1980 年的 102.2% 下降至 2021 年的 92.5%（图 1-2）。将各类食物按照能量统一换算后，能量自给率表现出下降趋势，由 93.6% 下降至 80.2%（表 1-3）。

表 1-2　1980—2021 年中国主要食物人均供给量

年份	人均供给量（千克 / 年）					
	粮食	食用油	蔬菜	水果	肉类	奶类
1980	337.8	3.6	53.5	6.6	12.0	1.2
1990	389.7	6.9	109.6	15.7	24.1	3.8
2000	360.2	10.5	344.3	48.2	47.2	6.8
2010	455.2	21.0	412.5	145.9	58.8	24.9
2020	560.6	26.6	522.3	202.0	60.5	37.2
2021	598.5	27.5	541.5	213.0	68.8	41.6

注：粮食包括谷物、薯类（5 千克鲜薯折算为 1 千克粮食）、杂豆和大豆。

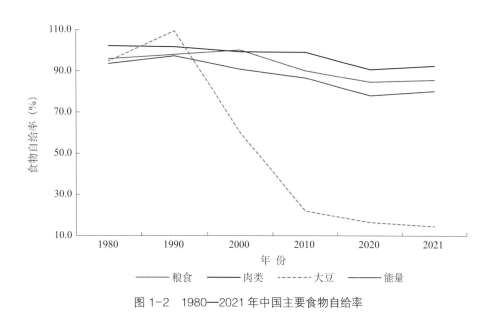

图 1-2　1980—2021 年中国主要食物自给率

表 1-3　1980—2021 年中国人均能量生产及供应情况

年份	自给率（%）	国内产量（千卡/天）	进口量（千卡/天）	总供给量（千卡/天）	饮食供给量（千卡/天）	其他供给量（工业用及饲用）（千卡/天）
1980	93.6	2 314.6	157.5	2 472.1	2 146.0	326.1
1994	97.3	2 891.2	79.8	2 971.0	2 504.0	467.0
2000	90.9	3 019.8	302.2	3 322.0	2 808.0	514.0
2010	86.6	3 401.4	526.1	3 927.5	3 044.0	883.5
2020	78.0	3 599.4	1 013.5	4 612.9	3 445.0	1 167.9
2021	80.2	3 772.3	929.9	4 702.2	3 548.0	1 154.2

（二）动物性产品消费快速增加，食物消费种类多样化

1. 口粮消费降中趋稳，杂粮消费减少

口粮（包括谷物、薯类及杂豆，其中薯类按照 5 千克鲜薯折 1 千克粮食计算）的年人均消费量由 1980 年的 174.8 千克增长到 1990 年的 202.9 千克，后缓慢下降并逐步趋于稳定，2021 年为 197.4 千克。其中，谷物的年人均消费量由 1980 年的

151.9 千克增长到 1990 年的 187.0 千克，增长了 23.2%，1990 年之后消费量缓慢下降至 2021 年的 184.4 千克，减少了 1.4%。谷物消费量趋于稳定，但是，薯类和杂豆的年人均消费量，分别由 1980 年的 89.5 千克和 5.0 千克下降到 2021 年的 59.1 千克和 1.2 千克，分别减少 30.4% 和 76.0%。由此可见，口粮消费呈现结构单一的趋势，有必要采取措施促进杂粮消费，从而满足人们日常营养健康的需求（图 1-3）。

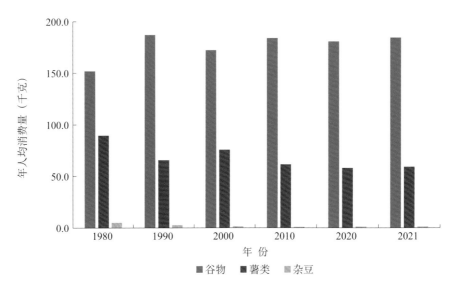

图 1-3　1980—2021 年谷物、薯类和杂豆的消费变化趋势

2. 动物产品消费不断增加，为优质蛋白质摄入提供保障

1980 年以来，我国动物产品消费呈现快速增长态势。肉类年人均消费量从 1980 年的 12.0 千克增加到 2021 年的 68.8 千克，增长量为 56.8 千克；其中，1980—2000 年肉类年人均消费量增长了 2.9 倍，2000—2021 年增长了 45.5%。蛋类年人均消费量从 1980 年的 2.5 千克增加到 2021 年的 21.8 千克，增长量为 19.3 千克；1980—2000 年蛋类年人均消费量增长了 5.2 倍，2000—2021 年涨幅放缓，增长了 41.6%。奶类年人均消费量从 1980 年的 0.9 千克增长到 2021 年的 37.0 千克，增长量为 36.1 千克；1980—2000 年奶类年人均消费量增长了 5.7 倍，2000—2021 年增长了 5 倍。水产品年人均消费量从 1980 年的 4.4 千克增长到 2021 年的

39.5 千克，增长量为 35.1 千克；1980—2000 年保持高速增长的态势，增长了 4.6 倍，2000—2021 年增长减缓，涨幅为 58.6%。总体上看，动物产品作为优质蛋白质来源，其消费保障了人们的营养健康需求（图 1-4）。

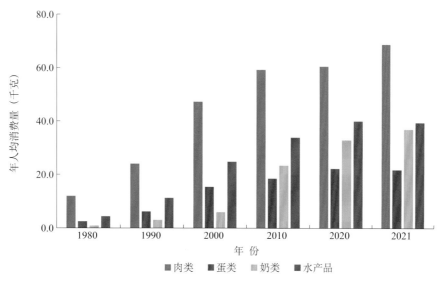

图 1-4　1980—2021 年动物产品的消费变化趋势

3. 水果、蔬菜消费持续快速增长，有效保障了微量营养素摄入

1980—2021 年，我国水果的年人均消费量从 5.9 千克增加到 180.0 千克，增长量为 174.1 千克；1980—2000 年快速增长，提高了 6.0 倍，2000—2021 年的增长速度虽有所下降，但仍增长了 3.4 倍。蔬菜的年人均消费量从 1980 年的 48.7 千克增加到 2021 年的 463.5 千克，增加了 414.8 千克；1980—2000 年保持高速增长的趋势，增长了 5.2 倍，2000—2021 年增长减缓，涨幅为 52.8%。水果、蔬菜富含膳食纤维、维生素和矿物质，为居民微量营养素摄入提供了重要保障（图 1-5）。

4. 植物油消费增势明显，食糖消费平稳波动且略有增长

植物油的年人均消费量呈现逐年增加的趋势，从 1980 年的 3.0 千克增加至 2021 年的 9.9 千克，增长量为 6.9 千克。其中，1980—2000 年的增速较快，增长了 1.0 倍，2000—2021 年的涨幅下降到 62.3%，但仍处于较高水平。目前，居民

食用植物油摄入量已超过推荐摄入量的上限，为预防油脂类摄入过多带来的超重肥胖问题，未来有必要采取相应措施引导居民适当减少植物油等油脂的消费（图 1-6）。

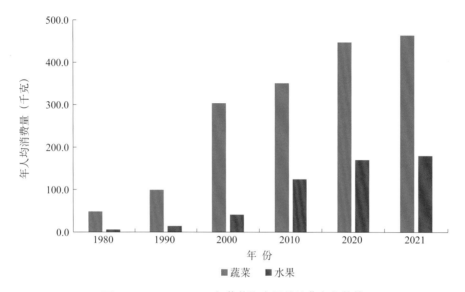

图 1-5 1980—2021 年蔬菜和水果的消费变化趋势

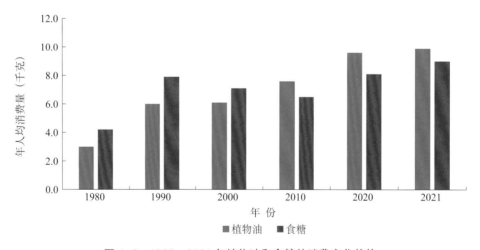

图 1-6 1980—2021 年植物油和食糖的消费变化趋势

食糖的年人均消费量由 1980 年的 4.2 千克增加到 2021 年的 9.0 千克，增长量为 4.8 千克。其中，1980—2000 年增长较快，增长了 69.0%，2000—2021 年增速放缓，增长了 26.8%。未来，为避免食糖摄入过多带来肥胖等慢性疾病问题，应引导居民适量消费（图 1-6）。

（三）居民营养大幅改善，能量供给充足

1. 居民能量、蛋白质及脂肪供给量持续增长

我国居民人均每日能量供给量由 1980 年的 2 146.2 千卡增加至 2021 年的 4 702.2 千卡，增长了 119.1%；同期，人均每日蛋白质及脂肪供给量分别由 53.4 克和 33.3 克增加至 102.8 克和 147.6 克，分别增长了 92.5% 和 343.2%（图 1-7）。人均脂肪供给量 2021 年比 1980 年增长超过 3 倍，涨幅最高。目前，人均能量及蛋白质供给量均高于《中国食物与营养发展纲要（2014—2020 年）》提出的 2020 年人均日推荐摄入量目标（能量 2 200～2 300 千卡，蛋白质 78 克）。

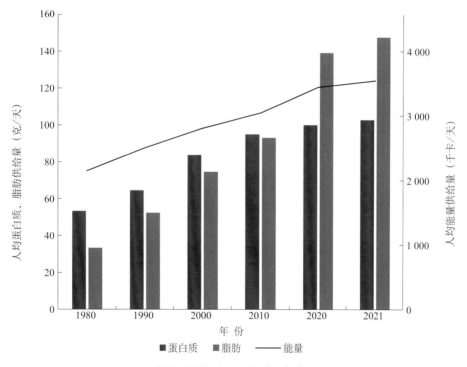

图 1-7　中国居民能量、蛋白质及脂肪人均供给量

碳水化合物提供能量占比由 1980 年的 76.1% 下降至 2021 年的 51.0%，下降了 25.1 个百分点；蛋白质和脂肪提供能量占比分别由 1980 年的 10.0% 和 14.0% 增加至 2021 年的 11.6% 和 37.4%，分别增长了 1.6 个百分点和 23.4 个百分点（表 1-4 和图 1-8）。

表 1-4　1980—2021 年中国居民能量供给营养素来源构成

年份	总能量		碳水化合物提供的能量		蛋白质提供的能量		脂肪提供的能量	
	供给量（千卡/天）	占比（%）	供给量（千卡/天）	占比（%）	供给量（千卡/天）	占比（%）	供给量（千卡/天）	占比（%）
1980	2 146.0	100.0	1 632.7	76.1	213.6	10.0	299.7	14.0
1990	2 504.0	100.0	1 774.0	70.8	258.4	10.3	471.6	18.8
2000	2 808.0	100.0	1 801.8	64.2	334.8	11.9	671.4	23.9
2010	3 045.0	100.0	1 827.1	60.0	380.0	12.5	837.9	27.5
2020	3 444.9	100.0	1 792.1	52.0	400.0	11.6	1 252.8	36.4
2021	3 547.8	100.0	1 808.2	51.0	411.2	11.6	1 328.4	37.4

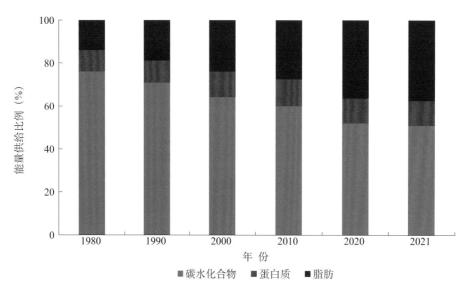

图 1-8　1980—2021 年中国居民能量供给营养素来源构成

2. 动物性食物来源的能量、蛋白质及脂肪快速增长

植物性食物来源的能量、蛋白质及脂肪的人均每日供给量分别由 1980 年的 1 981.0 千卡、46.5 克和 18.5 克增加至 2021 年的 2 821.2 千卡、60.5 克和 90.2 克，分别增长了 42.4%、30.1% 和 387.6%（表 1-5）。

动物性食物来源的能量、蛋白质及脂肪的人均每日供给量分别由 1980 年的 165.0 千卡、6.9 克和 14.8 克增加至 2021 年的 726.7 千卡、42.3 克和 57.4 克，分别增长了 3.4 倍、5.1 倍和 2.9 倍（表 1-5）。动物性食物能量及脂肪供给量的增加，可能引发营养供给不平衡，导致营养相关慢性病的发病风险增加。

1980—2021 年，植物性食物来源的能量人均每日供给量的增长量高于动物性食物，二者分别为 840.2 千卡、561.7 千卡，但植物性食物来源的蛋白质及脂肪人均每日供给量增长均低于动物性食物（表 1-5）。1980—2021 年，动物性食物提供能量、蛋白质及脂肪占比均有大幅提升，分别由 7.7%、12.9% 和 44.4% 增长到 20.5%、41.1% 和 38.9%。

表 1-5　1980—2021 年中国居民能量、蛋白质及脂肪不同食物来源供给

年份	植物性食物						动物性食物					
	能量		蛋白质		脂肪		能量		蛋白质		脂肪	
	供给量（千卡/天）	占比（%）	供给量（克/天）	占比（%）	供给量（克/天）	占比（%）	供给量（千卡/天）	占比（%）	供给量（克/天）	占比（%）	供给量（克/天）	占比（%）
1980	1 981.0	92.3	46.5	87.1	18.5	55.6	165.0	7.7	6.9	12.9	14.8	44.4
1990	2 216.0	88.5	51.4	79.6	27.2	51.9	288.0	11.5	13.2	20.4	25.2	48.1
2000	2 290.0	81.6	56.5	67.5	31.3	42.0	518.0	18.4	27.2	32.5	43.4	58.2
2010	2 358.0	77.4	57.9	61.0	37.3	39.6	687.0	22.6	37.1	39.1	55.9	59.4
2020	2 786.0	80.9	60.8	60.8	87.5	62.9	658.9	19.1	39.2	39.2	51.6	37.1
2021	2 821.2	79.5	60.5	62.3	90.2	61.1	726.7	20.5	42.3	41.1	57.4	38.9

3. 我国居民能量、蛋白质及脂肪供给总体超过世界平均水平

目前我国人均能量供给量，低于大部分欧美发达国家，高于印度、南非等发展中国家。按照 2019 年生产及供给水平计算，我国人均每日能量供给量为 3 347 千卡，低于美国、德国、加拿大、法国等国家人均能量供给量水平（3 532～3 862 千卡），与英国、俄罗斯、西班牙等国家水平相当（3 348～3 395 千卡），高于南非、

日本、印度等国（2 581～2 898 千卡）。我国人均每日蛋白质供给量，低于葡萄牙和美国等国（115.0～117.7 克），与大部分发达国家较为接近（104.2～109.7 克），但高于韩国、日本、南非和印度等国（64.9～99.0 克）。人均脂肪供给量同样低于大部分欧美发达国家，高于部分发展中国家。总体来看，我国居民能量、蛋白质及脂肪供给总体超过世界平均水平（表 1-6）。

表 1-6 2019 年不同国家人均能量、蛋白质及脂肪供给量

国家	能量人均供给量 （千卡 / 天）	蛋白质人均供给量 （克 / 天）	脂肪人均供给量 （克 / 天）
美国	3 862	115.0	180.1
德国	3 559	104.2	149.6
加拿大	3 539	108.6	156.0
法国	3 532	109.7	151.5
葡萄牙	3 458	117.7	140.1
韩国	3 453	99.0	123.5
澳大利亚	3 417	107.9	159.7
英国	3 395	106.2	138.7
俄罗斯	3 363	104.8	110.5
西班牙	3 348	108.5	154.7
中国	3 347	105.3	105.2
巴西	3 246	93.8	131.4
乌克兰	3 036	90.1	91.6
南非	2 898	79.8	87.5
日本	2 691	88.0	89.2
印度	2 581	64.9	59.8
世界平均	2 963	83.2	88.0

问题与挑战

（一）膳食不平衡，营养过剩和营养缺乏并存

1. 居民不健康生活方式仍然普遍存在

全球疾病负担研究显示，不合理膳食是中国疾病发生和死亡的主要原因。全谷物、深色蔬菜、水果、奶类、鱼虾类和大豆的摄入量依然低于推荐摄入量，我国仅有 20% 的消费者全谷物及杂粮摄入能达到推荐摄入量。高油高盐摄入仍普遍存在，含糖饮料消费逐年上升。《中国居民膳食指南科学研究报告（2021）》显示，相当数量中国人的心脏疾病、脑卒中和 2 型糖尿病死亡率与膳食因素有关。2017 年归因于膳食不合理的死亡人数为 310 万人，相比于 2012 年的 151 万人增加了约 1 倍。膳食不合理的诸多因素中，高钠摄入的膳食问题对心血管代谢死亡影响最大，2012 年占比 17.3%；高红肉摄入对心血管代谢死亡影响的占比增速最快，近 30 年占比增长了约 1.5 倍。全球知名医学杂志《柳叶刀》2019 年发布的"195 个国家和地区饮食结构造成的死亡率和疾病负担"研究显示，在饮食结构导致的死亡排行榜上，前三名分别为高钠摄入、全谷物摄入不足和水果摄入不足（图 2-1）。

2. 居民超重肥胖问题不断凸显

从科学膳食供能比的角度看，脂肪供能比上限为 30%。《中国居民营养与慢性疾病状况报告（2020）》显示，城乡居民的人均脂肪供能比均超过推荐上限，其中居民每标准人膳食脂肪供能比为 34.6%，城乡分别为 36.4% 和 33.2%，农村人口这一比例首次超过 30%。从人数上看，脂肪供能比超过 30.0% 的人数比例为 63.6%。居民超重肥胖问题不断凸显，慢性病患病、发病仍呈上升趋势。目前中国 18 岁及以上居民的超重肥胖率为 50.7%，其中超重率为 34.3%，肥胖率为 16.4%。

3. 微量营养素摄入不足问题仍然存在

近年来，我国居民维生素 A、铁、锌等微量营养素摄入情况有所改善，但隐性饥饿问题仍影响居民健康。《中国居民营养与慢性疾病状况报告（2020）》显示，

18 岁及以上居民低血清铁蛋白率为 13.3%，6～17 岁儿童与青少年为 11.2%，孕妇为 54.4%。2018 年 18 岁及以上居民的贫血率依然有 8.7%，孕妇则更高，达到 13.6%。18 岁及以上居民血清维生素 A 缺乏率（含边缘缺乏率，下同）为 4.7%，6～17 岁儿童与青少年为 15.7%，孕妇为 9.6%。

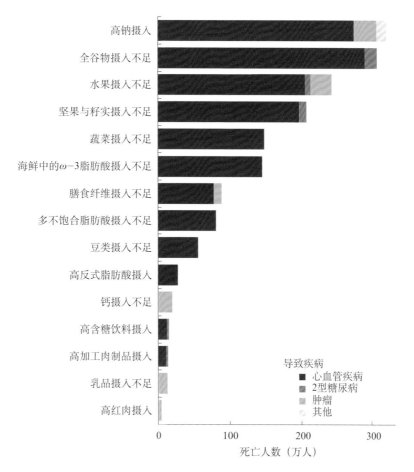

图 2-1　2017 年全球归因于个人饮食风险的死亡人数

（二）过度加工导致营养损失较大，全产业链食物损耗浪费严重

1. 过度加工导致主食营养损失较多

我们饮食传统里有着"食不厌精"的习惯，对大米、白面越来越追求"白、精、美"，面粉成了"雪花粉"，大米成了"亮精精"。精米、白面把谷物籽粒表皮和胚芽几乎全部去掉了，仅保留胚乳部分，造成谷物营养成分的极大损失。研

究表明，加工精度较高的面粉与全麦粉相比，蛋白质、维生素 B₁、维生素 B₂、烟酸、铁、钙、锌分别损失了 15%、83%、67%、50%、80%、50%、80%。对于稻谷而言，米糠虽然仅占稻谷质量的 5%～8%，却集中了稻谷 64% 的营养素。从加工副产品使用上看，主要用作饲料原料，少部分进入食品加工行业，国内对加工副产品利用很充分，虽然从数量上看损耗浪费不大，但过度加工造成的营养损失较大，长期食用精米白面有可能出现因维生素、矿物质等营养素缺乏造成的"隐性饥饿"，对身体健康有潜在风险。

2. 产业链前端食物损耗较大

据农业农村部食物与营养发展研究所调研，我国食物总体损耗率为 14.7%，略高于世界平均水平（13.8%）。分品种看，蔬菜、水果、水产品、粮食、肉类、奶类和蛋类损耗率分别为 25.9%、13.1%、8.1%、7.0%、6.6%、4.6% 和 3.4%。从环节上来看，农业生产、产后处理、贮藏、加工和流通环节损耗率分别为 4.3%、4.9%、2.6%、0.5% 和 2.3%，损耗主要发生在产业链前端，农业生产及产后处理的损耗量约占总损耗量的 63%，加工环节损耗率最低，平均为 0.5%（图 2-2）。按照 2021 年产量数据，我国食物损耗总量为 3.0 亿吨，折合成能量、蛋白质和脂肪分别为 164.7 万亿千卡（9.5%）、710 万吨（10.0%）和 253 万吨（7.3%）。

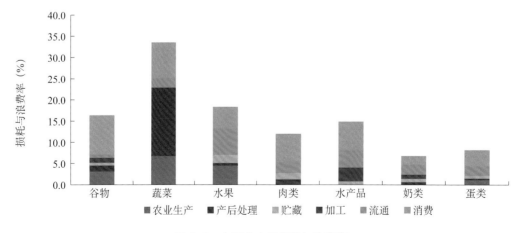

图 2-2 中国农产品损耗与浪费率

（数据来源：农业农村部食物与营养发展研究所动物食物与营养政策团队调研、
中国科学院地理科学与资源研究所成升魁团队调研）

3. 餐饮消费浪费严重

据中国科学院地理科学与资源研究所典型城市调研，受"面子文化"的影响，城市餐饮食物浪费严重，人均食物浪费量为 93 克／餐（以熟食计，下同），浪费率为 11.7%，商务宴请、大型聚会浪费比例更高。比较而言，家庭食物浪费相对有限，食物浪费率为 4.8%，家庭和餐馆加权平均食物浪费率约 8.0%。按照 2021 年产量数据，我国食物浪费总量为 1.6 亿吨，折合成能量、蛋白质、脂肪分别为 146.4 万亿千卡（8.4%）、569 万吨（8.1%）、241 万吨（7.0%）。

（三）科学饮食理念相对滞后，食物营养科普亟待加强

1. 食物营养认知转变相对滞后，很多人仍停留在"吃饱吃好"阶段

随着我国社会经济的不断发展，居民的生活水平日益提高，膳食结构发生了较大变化，但居民的食物营养认知没有及时转变，仍固守着温饱时代的高能量偏好与色香味体验，不重视饮食中的营养均衡。中国健康与营养调查（China Health and Nutrition Survey，CHNS）数据显示，2015 年，作为中国家庭膳食安排主导者的育龄妇女，其营养知识水平为 52%，老年人更低，仅 30.5%。即使在居民营养素养高于全国同期水平的上海市，2018 年仍有超过 50% 的市民不知母乳喂养的好处，同样比例的市民不了解吃大豆食品对身体健康的好处等。对于中老年人群，半数以上在选购包装食品时不注意生产日期、保质期、营养成分表和生产厂家等信息。部分富裕起来的人群仍然将大鱼大肉、厚油重酱、饮料快餐、高盐高糖食品作为"吃得好"的标志。快餐、外卖与预制菜行业迅速发展，营养健康标准亟须完善。2021 年，我国快餐业市场规模达 10 994 亿元，占中国餐饮业的 23.4%。居民外出就餐、点外卖、购买预制菜的比例逐渐上升。快餐在营养搭配、用油、用盐、用糖方面尚缺乏规范指导。

2. 科普引导渠道较乱，有效供给尚待提高

食物与营养知识的普及不够。一是食物营养科普工作的受重视程度不够，经

费投入不足，科普场馆和基地覆盖率较低，科普从业者的激励机制不健全，人才短缺。二是科普内容针对性不强，科普内容选择背离市场需求，经常忽视甚至不了解消费者的真实需求，往往偏重于狭义的科技内容，枯燥乏味，缺少针对性，与人们的实际饮食需求相距甚远。三是科普作品系统性较弱，科学合理专业性强、通俗易懂针对性强、容易操作实用性强的科普作品缺乏。大部分作品内容形式相对比较单一，吸引力和感染力有待进一步提升。

3. 会做饭的年轻人越来越少，迫切需要加强食育教育

当今社会，由于社会分工越来越细，生活压力越来越大，不会做饭的年轻人比比皆是。除时间优化分配的原因外，最主要的原因是在我国的传统教育体系中，缺乏对学生食物制作技能的培养和训练。科学网的一项调查显示，近六成大学生缺乏烹饪技能。无独有偶，美团外卖分析报告也指出"90 后"单身人群是点外卖的主力军，占比超 62%，其中 40% 的人不会做饭。总体来看，我国居民的饮食素养还有较大的提升空间，健康饮食技能还需要进一步夯实。

4. 食物宣传商业导向明显，网红主导传播模式

由于规范权威机构食物营养科普偏少，食品生产、流通等经营主体从自身利益出发，针对自己的产品，紧盯消费者的需求和知识盲点，广泛开展产品营销活动。这些经营主体虽然针对渠道、人群与食物品类的特征进行了细分和匹配，但有的在内容方面断章取义，选择性地片面夸大功效。更有个别网络平台，特别是自媒体，披着"科学实验、有图就是真相"的外衣，利用年轻人对网络名人的信任，进行危言耸听的宣传，制造热点，通过"吃播""带货"对消费者造成误导，损害正规食物营养科学引导工作的权威性和公信力。

（四）食物资源数据匮乏，缺乏监测评价标准

1. 食物资源家底不清

习近平总书记提出的大食物观，要求向森林要食物，向江河湖海要食物，向

设施农业要食物，向更丰富的生物资源拓展，向植物、动物与微生物要热量、要蛋白质。贯彻大食物观的首要困难是家底不清。

一是数据不清。目前，国家统计局公布的数据仅包括主要农产品宏观统计数据，缺乏小众特色食物数据，对特色新型小众食物的资源存量、分布、实际产能、消费结构等特征不清。二是食物资源开发利用的程度和范围不清。以植物性食物资源为例，由中国科学院植物研究所和中国科学院昆明植物研究所联合建设的中国植物主题数据库收集了 15.5 万余条植物数据，其中食用植物数据库数据记录不足 1 200 条。2021 年庄会富等发布的中国有用植物资源数据库，从各类志书、文献等提取出中国有用植物记录数 51 949 条，其中可食用的植物记录数 5 247 条（数据中含有重复记录，且包含用作调味品的植物以及用作食材加工后方可食用的植物等）。该套数据在现有食用植物资源数据中记录相对全面，但该套数据仅记录了可食用植物资源的名称（中文和拉丁文）、用途和分类等内容，未对这些食物资源的开发利用程度和应用范围进行梳理，无法为国家未来调整食物资源开发利用的战略布局提供基础数据支撑。三是营养特性不清。食物营养特征为制定营养政策，解决肥胖、隐性饥饿等营养不良问题提供基础支撑。我国长期以来主要关注食物的数量安全和质量安全，对营养安全的关注刚刚起步。现有食物成分表中的食物种类有限，只包含常规的宏量和微量营养素，缺乏功能性营养成分、风味物质和活性因子等数据。此外，现有食物成分表缺乏定期更新机制，数据更新缓慢，无法为营养政策和农业政策的调整提供重要支撑。

2. 食物资源营养品质监测与评价缺乏标准

一是品质监测体系不健全。现有监测体系重点关注农药与兽药残留、重金属、生物毒素、微生物等安全与卫生指标，忽视营养品质评价。二是食物营养评价处于起步阶段。现有评价指标不健全，评价方法不规范，缺少分等分级标准，难以有效规范市场，导致很多食物资源仍然难以从森林草原、海洋湖泊和边远地区走出来。三是缺乏定期监测工作机制和制度。在资源分布上，我国国土面积广阔，农业食物资源多样丰富，部分食物资源处于边远地区、山区和少数民族地区，种类、数量与营养特性十分复杂，目前也存在鱼目混珠的状况，比较混乱。在行政管理上，涉及农业农村部、自然资源部、国家卫生健康委员会、国家市场监督管理总局等不同部门，尚未建立定期监测机制，也缺少相应的法规制度。

3. 食物资源研究投入不足，科技创新能力薄弱

食物与国计民生和国民健康息息相关，但目前，我国对食物资源监测评价的科研投入不足，主要集中在粮食等重要农产品生产上。目前我国农业科技研发投入占比仅为 0.7% 左右，与发达国家 2% 以上的投入强度差距较大，传统农畜产品之外的特色食物开发利用获得的投入更为有限。受科技投入不足的影响，人才队伍、学科体系、平台条件建设相对滞后，严重制约了创新能力的提升。

向营养健康转型

（一）发展营养导向型农业，加快食物系统转型

发展营养导向型农业，是推动食物系统营养转型、支撑居民膳食结构优化和消除营养不良的重要举措，需要"以可持续发展为目标，以营养导向为理念，以资源禀赋为出发点"，重构农业产业链和食物价值链。

1. 加快农产品营养标准建设，指导动植物育种、种植养殖技术创新，推进营养导向型食物生产体系建设

针对食物生产存在的优质产品供给不足、微量营养素下降明显等严峻挑战，迫切需要转变理念，由"产量为主"转向"产量营养并重"。一是加快推进农产品营养标准体系建设，优先制定一批技术成熟、产业急需的示范性标准，引导协会、企业等各方主体积极参与标准建设，推动食物生产加快向营养转型。二是将营养品质纳入育种和生产的重要目标，加快构建包括营养品质、感官品质、加工品质在内的综合品质评价体系，培育更多高营养密度、优质专用的动植物新品种。三是加快研发一批营养导向的种植、养殖调控新技术，生产更多具有特定营养功能的优质农产品。

2. 提倡适度加工、精准加工，推动农产品加工减损增效，加快营养导向型食品加工体系建设

针对过度追求风味口感导致营养损失过多的突出问题，迫切需要革新理念，坚持"营养健康优先、兼顾美味口感"的指导思想，推动适度加工、精准加工与柔性制造。一是系统研究农产品全产业链营养品质变化规律，为适度、精准加工技术创新提供理论支撑。二是提升产地初加工和商品化处理水平，避免过度处理。引导企业合理确定小麦、稻谷等口粮品种加工精度，发展专用粉、全麦粉、专用米、糙米等新型健康产品。三是充分利用麦麸、米糠、果皮和果渣等开发植物油、膳食纤维、蛋白质制品等产品，提高食物综合利用效率。

3. 将营养导向融入所有政策，增加健康膳食的可负担性和可及性，加快推进营养导向型消费体系建设

针对居民膳食结构不合理、膳食理念不科学等突出问题，迫切需要优化完善消费引导政策体系。一是完善现有营养标签标识体系，改造提升预包装食品营养标签制度，大力推广食品正面包装（FOP）标签和生鲜农产品营养标识体系。二是要着力改善食物消费环境，创建营养健康食堂餐厅。针对高盐高油高糖食品，探索食品标识或税收等限制政策。三是在社会保护政策中明确营养内容，加强针对弱势群体的食物援助，如农村义务教育阶段学生营养改善计划等，要确保高营养品质和均衡搭配，增加健康饮食的可负担性和可获得性。

（二）打造第三口粮，提升主食多样性

食物多样是保障居民均衡膳食的基石。联合国粮食及农业组织将生物多样性作为粮食安全和营养的根本保障；五谷为养一直是中华饮食文明的重要内容。据2015—2017 年中国居民营养与健康状况监测数据，我国居民杂粮与薯类摄入量在谷薯类摄入量中的占比仅有 17.9%。由此可见，口粮品种过于集中，杂粮和全谷物摄入不足，既降低了主食多样性，带来了巨大的健康隐患，也给粮食安全带来了巨大压力。杂粮和全谷物是优化口粮结构、平衡膳食营养的最佳选择。杂粮品种众多，大多不与主粮争水争地，且 B 族维生素、膳食纤维、微量元素含量丰富，是优化口粮结构、改善营养供给的重要品种，具有明显的营养优势和不可替代性。与小麦、稻谷两大口粮品种相比，发展杂粮边际效应较高，只要努力，就会有明显成效。引导增加杂粮消费迫在眉睫、势在必行。教育消费者科学认识杂粮在实现健康膳食、均衡营养中的作用地位，培养消费习惯，增加杂粮主食，推动五谷杂粮回归居民餐桌主位，努力打造第三口粮，力争到 2035 年，杂粮与薯类摄入量占比翻一番，达到 35%。

1. 优化杂粮区域布局，构建适应居民营养健康需求的产业链，推动产业提质增效

一是因地制宜优化杂粮生产布局。根据全国《特色农产品优势区建设规划纲要》指导原则，在黄土高原区、内蒙古及长城沿线区、东北地区、西北风沙干旱区、太行山沿线区、西南石漠化区等，积极发展杂粮、杂豆和薯类种植。二是大力发展杂粮加工业，完善上下游产业链。推动传统杂粮食品的标准化规模化生产，通过"二产"带动"一产"和"三产"。探索推行产业链"链长制"等制度创新，建立涵盖育种推广专家以及生产、加工、贸易、流通、零售企业的对接平台，实现创新链与产业链深度衔接。三是大力提高种植效益，提高生产杂粮的积极性。探索杂粮产业优质优价实现机制，推动传统杂粮食品走出民间、走出主产区，走向全国大市场，扩大消费，进而提高农民种植效益。

2. 加大杂粮新品种选育和优质高产高效生产技术创新，提高优质原料供给水平

一是加大杂粮新品种选育与推广。以市场需求为导向，对现有品种的营养品质、加工品质、适口性等进行科学评价，筛选出优质专用、适口性好的品种。建立杂粮种子育繁推体系，着力解决"谁来育、谁来繁、谁来供、谁来推"职责不明确、管理不到位等方面问题，大力推动杂粮种业发展。二是加快优质高产高效生产技术创新。重点加强品质调控种植技术创新、轻简化专用农机装备创制、良种良法配套、农机农艺融合的技术集成模式和生产规范制定，提高生产效率和产品品质，提高优质原料供给水平。

3. 尽快突破杂粮生产加工调制关键技术，改善风味口感

粗杂粮产品不易煮熟、口感粗糙、不易消化吸收等问题是制约消费的重要因素。一是大力开发微粉化处理、低温烘焙、微波熟化等改善口感与蒸煮特性的现代食品加工技术，实现杂粮中酚类、多糖、脂类、植物甾醇等活性成分的保持与高效利用，把握加工精度、食用品质与活性保持的最佳平衡。二是引导企业针

对不同人群的膳食营养需求，进行"对症"的科学营养搭配，开发快熟杂粮伴侣、即食杂粮冲调代餐粉等杂粮产品和全谷物食品等，实现美味与营养健康深度融合。

（三）实施白肉增长计划，推动健康低碳饮食

以禽肉和水产品为代表的白肉具有脂肪含量较低、不饱和脂肪酸含量较高的特点，是健康优质蛋白质来源的首选，越来越受到消费者的青睐。2016 年，全球禽肉产量已经超过猪肉，成为全球第一大肉类产品；1990 年，美国禽肉产量超过牛肉，占肉类总产量的 37.6%，禽肉成为美国第一大肉类产品；2019 年，美国禽肉产量占比达 47.5%。禽肉产量快速增长的主要是因为其饲料转化率高，明显优于牛羊肉、猪肉等红肉产品，对资源环境压力显著小于其他肉类产品。此外，白肉摄入增加，可以有效减少脂肪摄入量，据《中国食物成分表》数据加权计算可知，每 100 克禽肉中含脂肪 9.4 克，比猪肉低 20.7 克。初步预测，2035 年我国居民肉类人均消费将达到 75 千克的峰值，在其他肉类产品保持不变的情况下，肉类消费增值部分由禽肉或水产品补充，在"碳中和、碳达峰"的发展目标下，兼顾居民营养健康和不过度增加资源环境压力等因素，具有重要意义，建议实施"白肉增长"战略。

1. 制定促进禽肉和水产品发展政策

将禽类和水产品发展放到养殖业中更加突出的位置，作为农业产业中优先发展的战略产业，加大养殖、屠宰加工、环境治理等方面支持力度。引导开发性、政策性金融机构加大对禽肉产业的支持，特别是利用好支农、支小再贷款和贷款贴息等政策，支持企业发展生产。

2. 加强家禽、水产繁育和养殖关键核心技术创新

在国家科技计划中，加大对家禽和水产养殖业的支持力度，聚焦品种繁育和推广应用，支持建立国家良种扩繁推广基地，引导种业企业与规模养殖场 / 塘建

立紧密的利益联结机制，增强禽类和水产品品种研发与转化能力。

3. 推动产业向规模化、标准化、智能化发展

以高标准养殖场 / 塘建设为抓手，提高禽肉和水产品生产过程中生物安全体系建设，提高智能化设施设备利用水平，提升禽类和水产品的现代化养殖水平，推动产业持续健康发展。加强关于白肉安全、营养、健康的科普，建立消费者对白肉产品的品质信任及动物性食物健康消费理念。

（四）依靠科技减少损耗，厉行节约杜绝浪费

我国是农业和人口大国，水土资源有限，食物增产难度越来越大，减少食物损耗与浪费对于保障我国粮食安全和食物系统可持续发展尤为重要。2021 年，我国食物损耗和浪费率合计 22.7%，初步估算约有一半的减损空间，即 11.35 个百分点，可节约 2.3 亿吨食物，折合成热量为 155.7 万亿千卡，可满足 1.9 亿人 1 年的营养需求，减少 2.5 亿亩耕地资源使用、1.5 亿立方米水资源消耗和 1.6 亿吨温室气体排放。

1. 加大投入，强化食物减损的基础设施与科技支撑

提高收割、储藏、分割等环节的机械化、智能化水平，推广先进冷链设备应用，提高产地冷藏保鲜处理比重，加快补齐农产品冷链产地"最前一公里"短板；加快推进食物减损关键环节、重点领域标准研制，推动先进技术、工艺、设备等及时应用于食物减损实践。

2. 缩短食物运输里程，减少生鲜农产品流通损耗

随着农业生产逐渐向优势产区集中，"南菜（果）北运"等现象日益突出，流通环节多、距离长造成大量食物损耗。鼓励大中城市利用近郊农业土地，加大蔬菜等非耐贮运生鲜农产品基地建设力度，确保自给率至少在 30% 以上。加强主产区与重要城市重点地区协调配合，合理设置配送半径，提高农产品流通效率，

缩短食物配送里程，提高食物系统供给效率与韧性。

3. 多举并用，大力反对食物浪费

加快推动《中华人民共和国反食品浪费法》贯彻实施，进一步细化配套规定，尽快制定完善相关配套规定，建立反食品浪费的长效机制。遏制餐饮行业食品浪费，鼓励"分餐制""小份餐"，支持餐饮企业对消费者的浪费行为适当加收费用。加强反食品浪费宣传教育，积极倡导文明、健康、科学的饮食文化，增强全社会的反食品浪费意识，营造节约光荣、浪费可耻的社会氛围。

（五）从娃娃和掌勺人抓起，推进健康饮食教育

健康饮食教育既关乎个体身体健康，也关乎一个民族饮食文化的传承，以及人类群体的可持续发展。健康饮食教育是一个系统工程，进校园、进家庭是两个关键环节。

1. 促进食育进校园，把食育纳入幼儿园、中小学教学体系

食育是智育的前提和基础，是提升儿童、青少年乃至全民营养水平的首选策略。把食育放在"德智体美劳"同等重要的位置，将食育纳入幼儿园、中小学教学体系。系统性地将饮食知识和良好的饮食习惯，纳入学龄前教育，并以食物为载体，进行道德、文化、营养科学和可持续发展意识的引导与培养。中小学要加大食育教材的编写和师资培训，重点加强教师食物营养知识与素养的提升，充分发挥教师群体在食育中的主体地位和积极性。在幼儿园、中小学食堂配备专职营养师，配制符合学生生长发育阶段需求的营养餐，充分发挥学生食堂在营养教育中的示范作用，提高学生食物营养素养。

2. 促进食育进家庭，发挥掌勺人在食育中的主导地位

鉴于家庭食育途径多、成本低、涉及面广，已被多个国家政府、卫生部门和营养界作为改善儿童、青少年及家庭营养状况的主要手段。积极推进家庭食育，

倡导居家就餐，开办掌勺人食育课堂，提升食物营养知识技能。各级食物营养科研机构和社会团体积极开展家庭食育相关模式研究、交流、引导与实践。在规范快餐健康发展的同时，积极倡导家庭慢食。

3. 加强主流科普团队培养，推动传播格局重构

各级政府要充分认识营养科普宣传对健康中国建设的重要意义，将营养科普作为重要战略措施，加大投入力度。主流媒体、各级食物营养相关科研院所、高等院校、学会协会等单位要主动承担食物营养科普职责，创新传播方式，作为主渠道发挥其在食物营养科普中的主导作用。逐步完善食物与营养科普奖励制度，鼓励食物营养领域科研工作者和行业从业人员积极从事科普工作。国家食物与营养咨询委员会等权威食物营养智库要进一步完善相关新媒体平台建设，加大科普宣传与实践基地建设力度。科普行业应加强自律和监管，相关部门应加大对宣扬伪科学的惩处力度。

（六）开展食物资源普查，构建食物监测评价体系

按照大食物观的要求，目前我国食物营养品质监测评价还缺乏科学的标准，科技条件建设滞后，难以支撑食物资源的高效开发利用。因此，需要尽快建立食物资源及其营养特征的数据库与监测评价体系。

1. 开展食物资源监测

建立覆盖各区域各品类的食物监测体系，规范监测指标和方法，应用多源多模态数据融合认知计算技术、基础农产品标准知识图谱、数据库技术、多源气象数据技术、区块链技术、遥感技术、电子围栏标识技术等，充分整合各部门现有食物数据资源，建立食物资源开发利用数据库和食物营养品质监测数据库。

2. 开展特色食物资源的品质特性评价

围绕食物资源的营养组分、感官特性和活性因子，采用蛋白质组学、代谢组

学和食品组学技术对食物资源的特性进行高通量筛查识别，建立基于产地特征的多维评价方法，鉴定不同产地、品种和品质的食物资源，开发地理标志产品，制定分等分级标准，精准发挥不同食物资源的独特作用和营养健康价值。

3. 加强食物资源基础研究、技术创新和示范利用

建设食物资源监测与营养评价国家重点实验室，加大食物资源创新平台建设力度，建立食物资源评价的学科体系、人才培养体系。推动食物资源产业示范与发展，打造产业示范园区，强化信息示范，发挥好大数据、人工智能、云计算的重要作用，为增加食物多样性、营养多样性、生态多样性提供重要科技支撑。

参考文献

艾媒数据中心，2022. 餐饮行业数据分析：中国男性网民食用中式快餐频率与女性不同［EB/OL］. 艾媒网. https://www.iimedia.cn/c1061/84785.html.

餐饮新纪元，2020. 90后单身人群是点外卖的主力军占比超62%，其中40%的人不会做饭［EB/OL］.［2021-09-12］. https://www.163.com/dy/article/FGD8OHUK0519DCKC.html.

陈萌山，2021. 发展营养导向型农业建设健康中国［J］. 农村工作通讯（7）：21-23.

陈思佳，沈欣，郭若宜，等，2020. 亲子健康饮食教育模式对学龄前儿童早餐质量的影响［J］. 中国学校卫生，41（5）：769-771.

程蓓，2019. 食育的中国之策——基于日美两国的经验［J］. 中国德育（4）：14-18.

樊晓莉，孙桂菊，2022. 中国育龄女性膳食营养知识水平变化趋势及影响因素分析［J］. 中国公共卫生，38（6）：787-791.

顾锦春，范含信，2022. 乡村振兴背景下加强农村中学健康饮食教育的思考［J］. 现代农村科技（9）：93-95.

国家发展和改革委员会，农业农村部，国家林业和草原局，2022. 特色农产品优势区建设规划纲要［EB/OL］.［2022-09-12］. http://www.gov.cn/xinwen/2017-10/31/content_5235803.htm.

国家统计局，2021. 2021中国统计年鉴［M］. 北京：中国统计出版社.

国家卫生健康委疾病预防控制局，2021. 中国居民营养与慢性病状况报告（2020年）［M］. 北京：人民卫生出版社.

韩凤芹，周孝，史卫，等，2018. 我国财政科普投入及其效果评价［J］. 财政科学，36（12）：19-36.

黄家章，卢士军，姚远，等，2020. 基于文献计量的国际营养导向型农业研究进展可视化分析［J］. 中国农业科技导报，22（9）：11-21.

金妍，2022. 新媒体视野下科普传播模式及发展策略［J］. 中国报业（2）：90-91.

联合国粮食及农业组织，2019. 营养导向型农业与食物系统：干预措施［M］. 孙君茂，黄家章，卢士军，译. 北京：中国农业科学技术出版社.

卢士军，黄家章，吴鸣，等，2019. 营养导向型农业的概念、发展与启示［J］. 中国农业科学，52（18）：3083-3088.

马冠生，张曼，2019. 儿童饮食行为调查：经常吃快餐、喝饮料危害儿童健康［EB/OL］.［2021-09-12］. https://zhuanlan.zhihu.com/p/82106526.

农业农村部市场预警专家委员会，2020. 中国农业展望报告2020—2029［M］. 北京：中国农业科学技术出版社.

农业农村部市场预警专家委员会，2021. 中国农业展望报告 2021—2030［M］. 北京：中国农业科学技术出版社.

农业农村部市场预警专家委员会，2022. 中国农业展望报告 2022—2031［M］. 北京：中国农业科学技术出版社.

孙君茂，卢士军，江晓波，等，2019. 营养导向型农业国内外政策规划与启示［J］. 中国农业科学，52（18）：3089-3096.

唐洪涛，夏蕊，孙学安，等，2020. 家庭教育的重要一环：食育［J］. 中国校外教育（8）：1-2.

唐闻佳，2019. 超半数市民不知母乳喂养能让婴儿少生病，上海首发"健康素养 72 条"补常识短板［EB/OL］.［2021-09-12］. https://wenhui.whb.cn/third/baidu/201903/27/252 246.html.

王文月，臧明伍，张辉，等，2022. 我国食品科技创新力量布局现状与发展建议［J］. 食品科学，43（13）：336-341.

王瑜，黄程佳，2016. 我国幼儿食育必要性及其促进策略［J］. 学前理论教育，32（4）：15-19.

杨舒，2022. 新时代推进科普工作系统布局已形成——专家解读《关于新时代进一步加强科学技术普及工作的意见》［N/OL］. 光明日报.［2021-09-12］. https://share.gmw.cn/news/2022-09/06/content_36004950.htm.

中共中央办公厅，2022. 关于新时期进一步加强科学技术普及工作的意见［EB/OL］.［2022-09-12］. https://www.ncsti.gov.cn/zcfg/zcwj/202209/t20220905_96313.html.

中国疾病预防控制中心营养与健康所，2019. 中国食物成分表：标准版［M］. 6 版. 北京：北京大学医学出版社.

中国营养学会，2022. 中国居民膳食指南［M］. 北京：人民卫生出版社.

中研普华研究院，2021. 2022—2027 年版快餐产品入市调查研究报告［EB/OL］.［2021-09-12］https://3g.163.com/dy/article/HCN7MHDR0518H9Q1.html.

诸葛卫东，张一婧，傅一程，2020. 由奖励制度看日本科普策略与实践的发展方向［J］. 自然辩证法通讯，42（11）：101-110.

庄会富，王亚楠，王趁，等，2021. 中国有用植物资源数据库［J/OL］. 中国科学数据.［2021-09-12］. DOI: 10.11922/csdata.2021.0006.zh.

GBD 2017 Diet Collaborators，2019. Health effects of dietary risks in 195 countries，1990—2017: A systematic analysis for the Global Burden of Disease Study 2017［J］. The Lancet，393（10184）：1958-1972.

KIRK D，CATAL C，TEKINERDOGAN B，2021. Precision nutrition: A systematic literature review［J］. Computers in Biology and Medicine，133: 104365.

XUE L，LIU X，LU S，et al.，2021. China's food loss and waste embodies increasing environmental impacts［J］. Nature Food，2（7）：519-528.

附录 1 1980—2021 年中国各类食物产量

1980—2021 年中国各类食物产量

（单位：万吨）

年份	粮食	谷物	薯类	杂豆	蔬菜	水果	肉类	奶	蛋	水产品	大豆	坚果	糖	油
1980	32 055.5	27 719.0	15 870.0	670.0*	5 316.0*	679.3	1 205.4	114.1	280.0*	449.7	794.0	360.0	349.4	331.7*
1985	37 910.8	33 707.2	14 362.5	550.0*	9 277.5*	1 163.9	1 926.5	249.9	534.7	705.2	1 050.0	666.4	725.6	524.0*
1990	44 624.3	40 169.0	13 018.0	612.0*	12 910.1*	1 874.4	2 857.0	415.7	794.6	1 427.3	1 100.0	636.8	865.7	592.2*
1995	46 661.8	41 611.6	13 716.5	437.3	25 726.7	4 214.6	5 260.1	576.4	1 676.7	2 953.0	1 350.2	1 023.5	952.8	778.8*
2000	46 217.5	40 522.4	16 313.0	469.1	44 467.9	6 226.1	6 013.9	827.4	2 182.0	3 706.2	1 540.9	1 443.7	916.2	1 135.6*
2005	48 402.2	42 776.0	18 426.0	522.9	56 451.5	16 120.1	6 938.9	2 753.4	2 438.1	4 419.9	1 634.8	1 434.2	1 134.2	1 570.0*
2006	49 804.2	45 099.2	17 342.5	495.5	53 953.1	17 102	7 099.9	2 944.6	2 424.0	4 583.6	1 508.2	1 288.7	1 255.2	1 624.4*
2007	50 413.9	45 963.0	13 506.5	429.8	57 537.8	17 659.4	6 916.4	2 947.1	2 546.7	4 747.5	1 279.3	1 381.5	1 449.9	1 591.1*
2008	53 434.3	48 569.4	13 709.0	451.0	58 669.2	18 279.1	7 370.9	3 010.6	2 699.6	4 895.6	1 570.9	1 463.5	1 560.7	1 675.0*
2009	53 940.9	49 243.3	14 215.0	382.2	59 139.5	19 093.7	7 706.7	2 995.1	2 751.9	5 116.4	1 522.4	1 460.4	1 409.6	1 838.3*
2010	55 911.3	51 196.7	13 964.5	330.8	57 264.9	20 095.4	7 993.6	3 038.9	2 776.9	5 373.0	1 541.0	1 513.6	1 356.4	1 928.8*

续表

年份	粮食	谷物	薯类	杂豆	蔬菜	水果	肉类	奶	蛋	水产品	大豆	坚果	糖	油
2011	58 849.3	54 061.7	14 213.5	375.5	59 766.6	21 018.6	8 023.0	3 109.9	2 830.4	5 603.2	1 487.9	1 530.2	1 399.6	1 999.2*
2012	61 222.6	56 659.0	14 621.5	337.0	61 624.5	22 091.5	8 471.1	3 174.9	2 885.4	5 502.1	1 343.6	1 579.2	1 494.2	2 118.3*
2013	63 048.2	58 650.4	14 415.0	301.7	63 198.0	22 748.1	8 632.8	3 000.8	2 905.5	5 744.2	1 240.7	1 610.9	1 506.6	2 103.9*
2014	63 964.8	59 601.5	14 277.0	395.9	64 948.7	23 302.6	8 817.9	3 159.9	2 930.3	6 001.9	1 268.6	1 590.1	1 450.6	2 261.3*
2015	66 060.3	61 818.4	13 994.0	275.8	66 425.1	24 524.6	8 749.5	3 179.8	3 046.1	6 211.0	1 236.7	1 596.1	1 345.8	2 392.0*
2016	66 043.5	61 666.6	13 646.5	291.2	67 434.2	24 405.2	8 628.3	3 064.0	3 160.5	6 379.5	1 359.6	1 636.1	1 341.1	2 289.9*
2017	66 160.7	61 620.5	13 631.5	313.4	69 192.7	25 241.9	8 654.4	3 038.6	3 096.3	6 445.3	1 528.3	1 709.2	1 365.5	2 413.7*
2018	65 789.2	61 003.6	13 993.0	323.6	70 346.7	25 688.4	8 624.6	3 074.6	3 128.3	6 457.7	1 596.7	1 733.2	1 432.5	2 466.4*
2019	66 384.3	61 369.7	14 327.0	322.7	72 102.6	27 400.8	7 758.8	3 201.2	3 309.0	6 480.4	1 809.2	1 752.0	1 460.3	2 491.0**
2020	66 949.2	61 674.3	14 413.5	327.3	74 912.9	28 692.4	7 748.4	3 440.1	3 467.8	6 549.0	1 960.2	1 799.3	1 441.7	2 787.0**
2021	68 284.8	63 275.7	14 937.0	325.5**	77 548.8	29 970.2	8 990.0	3 682.7	3 408.8	6 463.7	1 640.0*	1 830.8	1 374.5	2 855.0**

数据来源：未标*数据来源于 1981—2021 年《中国统计年鉴》；标*数据来源于 FAO 食物平衡表；标**数据未源于《中国农业展望报告》。

附录 2 2021 年国内外食物与营养领域大事记

2021 年，新冠疫情席卷全球，对全球健康产生重大影响。针对此状况，国际上普遍采取措施改善营养状况，倡导食物系统转型以满足可持续发展、健康需求，以及实现全球范围内零饥饿。国内食物营养领域的工作主要聚焦于粮食安全、粮食减损、粮食系统和食物营养发展纲要等方面，反映出当我国食物数量安全基本得到保障后，伴随居民生活水平的提升和消费结构的升级，确保食物质量安全成为食物安全战略的现实高层次需求。本部分主要对具有代表性的典型事件进行回顾性梳理。

1 月 4 日，党的十九届五中全会审议通过《中共中央关于制定国民经济和社会发展第十四个五年规划和二〇三五年远景目标的建议》。同时，2021 年中央一号文件中，粮食安全问题被放于突出位置。提出牢牢守住保障国家粮食安全和不发生规模性返贫两条底线。推动经济社会平稳健康发展，必须着眼国家重大战略需要，稳住农业基本盘、做好"三农"工作，接续全面推进乡村振兴。2021 年，农业供给侧结构性改革深入推进，粮食播种面积保持稳定、产量达到 1.3 万亿斤以上，生猪产业平稳发展，农产品质量和食品安全水平进一步提高，农民收入增长继续快于城镇居民，脱贫攻坚成果持续巩固。

1 月 12 日，世界卫生组织发布《制定和实施促进健康饮食的公共食品采购和服务政策的行动框架》，概述了如何制定（或加强）、实施、评估健康的公共食品采购和服务政策，以及如何评价其有效性，供国家或区域、省和市一级相关政府决策者或方案管理人员使用。

2 月 10 日，联合国儿童基金会发布《关于预防儿童和青少年超重和肥胖的方案指南》，就如何调整方案编制和国家支助工作以应对不断变化的营养不良状况向各国提供战略指导，包括重点关注改善儿童食品环境的监管行动。

2 月 25 日，《中国居民膳食指南科学研究报告（2021）》正式发布。该报告内容包括我国居民膳食与营养健康现况及问题分析、膳食与健康研究的新证据、与主要健康结局风险降低相关的膳食因素，以及世界各国膳食指南关键内容推荐，助力促进我国居民合理膳食。

4 月 26 日，由农业农村部主办、中国农业科学院承办的国家粮食安全与可持续发展对话会在北京召开。会议响应联合国世界粮食峰会号召，以"推动可持续发展，保障国家粮食安全"为主题，在国家范围内召集粮食系统各个利益相关方开展对话，围绕中国粮食系统转型与政策支持、粮食生产与可持续发展、粮食减损与冲击应对、城乡居民的粮食安全与公平生计、可持续的食物消费 5 个议题进行专题报告和开放讨论，深入探讨中国粮食安全和农业可持续发展路径。

5 月 4 日，联合国粮食及农业组织发布《2022 年全球粮食危机报告》。该报告显示，2021 年有 53 个国家或地区约 1.93 亿人经历粮食危机，粮食不安全程度比 2020 年增加近 4 000 万人，创历史新高。造成粮食不安全状况加剧的主要原因是冲突、极端天气和经济危机。

5 月 6 日，《精准营养白皮书——精准营养研究与产业转化趋势》发布。该白皮书系统总结了国内外精准营养科研前沿和应用现状，深入分析了未来科研、行业面临的机遇与挑战，聚焦产学研融合，提供精准营养解决方案的产业转化思路，助力构建有活力的产业生态。

5 月 11 日，《健康谷物白皮书》发布。该白皮书对健康谷物摄入模式及消费现状等进行了系统的分析阐述，旨在引导消费者优化谷物摄入结构，增加全谷物消费，助力实现"健康中国 2030"可持续发展目标。

5 月 15 日，全民营养周暨"5·20"中国学生营养日活动在北京启动。活动聚焦"平衡 / 合理膳食"，旨在提倡营养配餐，推进健康家庭等建设，推动国民健康饮食习惯的形成和巩固，将健康中国合理膳食行动落到实处，在全社会形成营养、健康、不浪费的生活方式。

5 月 18 日，国家食物与营养咨询委员会召开年度工作会议，聚焦新纲要，研讨新发展，构建新格局，助力提振新冠疫情后的食物营养改善。农业农村部食物与营养发展研究所作为牵头编制单位，组织专家对《中国食物与营养发展纲要（2021—2035 年）》（送审稿）进行论证。该纲要的编制将对推动我国农业食物生产、城乡居民膳食结构转型升级、全面建设健康中国具有纲领性指导作用。

5 月 31 日，《2021 中国白领女性膳食健康白皮书》发布。该白皮书主要分析了我国城市 18～49 岁女性的食物与营养素摄入状况和膳食结构，以发现其目前存在的膳食与营养问题，并有针对性地提出具体改善策略与建议，促进其营养与健康。

6 月 20 日至 8 月 20 日，由农业农村部食物与营养发展研究所与联合国儿童基金会联合主办的中国青少年粮食系统主题对话会在成都等六地举办，就中国粮食系统的现状和发展开展了青少年对话。该对话会是我国响应联合国粮食系统峰会前期系列活动之一。对话会的举办，向全球传递了中国青少年对未来食物系统构建的观点，为今后建立更健康、更包容和更可持续的粮食系统贡献了中国青少年的智慧和力量。

7 月 21 日，《中国儿童青少年食物营养发展现状及对策》报告发布。该报告从营养状况、膳食营养摄入情况、食物消费问题 3 个方面分析了中国儿童与青少年食物营养发展现状，并据此提出了优化膳食结构、推广营养强化农产品等 7 项对策建议，对促进我国儿童与青少年营养改善和健康发展具有重要意义。

9 月 9—11 日，国际粮食减损大会在济南举办。在此期间，《国际粮食减损济南倡议》发布，向世界发出中国"粮"言，实现粮食减损、粮食安全的目标。作为全人类的共同命题，粮食安全是世界和平与可持续发展的重要保障。

9 月 23 日，首届联合国粮食系统峰会成功举办。利用粮食系统与营养不良、气候变化、贫困等全球挑战的相互关联性，推动 17 个可持续发展目标取得进展。旨在使所有人能够利用食物系统的力量从新冠疫情中复苏，使生产生活重回正轨。峰会上，有 165 个成员国发言，阐述了在国家和全球范围内推进食物系统

2030 议程的重要性，呼吁国际和区域合作，并使受到新冠疫情冲击的经济得以复苏，确保粮食安全、消除饥饿和营养改善的承诺实现。所有食物系统参与者都作出了大胆承诺，包括一些政府和其他合作伙伴作出重大财政承诺，以支持国内和国际食物系统的变革行动，并就改善营养和消除饥饿提出更加具体的举措。在多方的承诺下，出现了若干多方利益相关方的倡议和联盟，以支持落实国家和区域食物系统转型，包括关注零饥饿、健康饮食、学校供餐、减少食物浪费，此外，还发布了其他方面的多方利益相关者公告。

9 月 25 日，全球营养改善运动 3.0 在中亚和南亚地区正式启动。全球营养改善运动（Scaling Up Nutrition Movement，SUN 运动）已经覆盖了 65 个国家和 4 个印度州，在国家营养方面取得了重大进展，同时也在推动全球营养目标的进展方面发挥了关键作用。作为联合国粮食系统峰会的一部分，53 个成员国举办了对话，旨在加速建设粮食系统。此外，60 个成员国参加了东京营养促进增长峰会，并向营养问责框架提交了具体、可衡量的承诺。2021 年是全球营养改善运动的标志性"过渡与进步"时间节点之一。全球营养改善运动战略 3.0（2021—2025）启动，标志着该倡议第三阶段的开始，在众多成员国举办了相关活动。同时，全球营养改善运动秘书处进行了重组，以满足成员不断发展和进步的需求，成立了资源调动小组、战略咨询团队、融资能力发展平台。

10 月 21 日，联合国粮食及农业组织、国际农业发展基金和世界粮食计划署在欧洲联盟的财政支持下，共同启动了《促进粮食安全、改善营养和可持续农业的性别变革方法联合方案》。通过解决性别问题的根源实现可持续农业。在变革过程中赋予妇女权利并实现两性平等，来改善营养状况和粮食安全问题。

10 月 30—31 日，联合国粮食及农业组织在二十国集团领导人峰会上发表了《关于粮食安全、营养和粮食体系的马泰拉宣言》，呼吁国际社会共同建设有包容性和韧性的粮食系统，保证所有人获得充足营养，助力非洲国家早日实现"零饥饿"目标。

10 月 31 日至 11 月 13 日，英国在格拉斯哥主办了第二十六届联合国气候变化大会。近 200 个国家齐聚英国，承诺对气候变化采取行动，并制定《格拉斯哥气候公约》，以保持 1.5℃的生命力，最终完成《巴黎协定》中尚未完成的内容。联合国营养署将与一些行动者合作，强调食品和营养在缓解气候变化方面的关键作用，以及将营养纳入气候谈判的必要性。

11 月 23 日，全球营养领域专家联合撰写的《2021 年全球营养报告》发布。该报告分析了不良饮食对健康和地球的影响，评估了营养融资前景，概述了营养承诺的进展情况。该报告指出，尽管全球营养状况取得一些进展，但饮食没有更加健康，对环境的要求也越来越高，而不可接受的营养不良状况仍然存在。建议在财政投资、饮食和营养不良、问责制 3 个关键领域采取行动。

12 月 7—8 日，东京营养促进增长峰会举办。该次峰会召开于联合国营养行动十年的中期，距离实现世界卫生大会关于孕产妇、婴儿和幼儿营养的目标只剩下 5 年时间，距离实现可持续发展目标还有 10 年时间。此次峰会确定了 3 个核心领域：使营养成为全民健康保险的组成部分；建立促进健康饮食和营养、确保生产者生计和气候智能的粮食系统；在脆弱和受冲突影响的背景下有效解决营养不良。另外，在这些核心领域形成了新的共同目标，包括促进数据驱动问责制和确保推动营养融资创新，以此支持联合国营养行动十年和可持续发展目标。

12 月 29 日，《中国营养学会　膳食纤维专家共识》正式发布。该共识的发布将为《中国居民膳食营养素参考摄入量（DRIs）》以及相关法规中关于膳食纤维条款的修订提供基础资料，科学指导食品企业理解和应用膳食纤维。

1

From eating-full to eating-well

1.1 Food production has increased significantly, and the supply is sufficient

1.1.1 The grain output has remained above 650 million tons, and other foods continued to grow

Since the reform and opening-up, food production in China has steadily increased, ensuring the supply of rations. The grain production in China is increasing year by year, which was 682.848 million tons in 2021, and it has increased by 1.1 times from 320.555 million tons in 1980. The "Vegetable basket" (non-grain food supply) has been continuously enriched, and the output of vegetables, fruits, meat, eggs and milk has increased rapidly. In 2021, the output of vegetables and fruits reached 775.488 million tons and 299.702 million tons, up 14.0 times and 43.0 times respectively over 1980. The output of meat, eggs, milk and aquatic products was 89.900 million tons, 34.088 million tons, 36.827 million tons, and 64.637 million tons, which were increased by 6.5 times, 11.0 times, 31.3 times, and 13.4 times than that of 1980, respectively. The growth rates of fruit and milk were the fastest, which increased by more than 30 times. The oil-bearing crops and sugar have continuously increased. The oil-bearing crops increased from 7.691 million tons to 35.864 million tons, with a growth of 3.7 times. The edible vegetable oil increased from 3.317 million tons in 1980 to 28.55 million tons in 2021, with an increase of 7.6 times. Sugar increased from 3.494 million tons in 1980 to 13.745 million tons in 2021, with an increase of nearly 3 times (Figure 1-1).

1.1.2 The import of oil-bearing crops, oil products, milk and feed grain has increased rapidly after 2000

From 1980 to 2000, it changed from net grain import of 11.837 million tons to net grain export of 1.023 million tons in China (Table 1-1). The net exports of fruits and vegetables increased to 566,000 tons and 3,805,000 tons respectively, increased

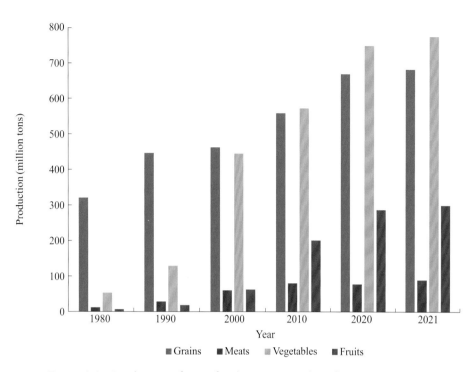

Figure 1-1   Production of main food varieties in China from 1980 to 2021

by 1.2 times and 6.8 times. The net export of eggs first decreased and then increased, fluctuating between 38,000 and 68,000 tons. The net oil-bearing crops export of 115,000 tons changed to a net import of 2.308 million tons. The net import of edible vegetable oil increased to 2.044 million tons, with an increase of 10.2 times. The net import of sugar reduced to 1.57 million tons, down by 76.7%. The net import of meat reached 290,000 tons. The net import of milk increased to 401,000 tons, with an increase of 12.8 times. The net import of aquatic products increased to 4.59 million tons, with an increase of 167.2 times.

In 2000, since China joined WTO, the import of soybean, palm oil, and feed grains has increased rapidly. In 2021, the net grain import increased to 162.65 million tons, of which soybean import reached about 100 million tons. The net export of fruits began to decline after reaching a peak in 2010, which changed into net import for the first time in 2021, with a net import of 1.12 million tons. The net export of vegetables increased to 10.62 million tons in 2021, with an increase of 1.8 times. The net import of oil-bearing crops reached 5.532 million tons. The net import of edible vegetable oil reached 10.27 million tons, with an increase of 4.0 times. The net sugar import reached 6.21 million tons, with an increase of 3.0 times. The net import of meat reached 7.308 million tons, which increased by 24.2 times. The net import of milk increased to 21.95 million tons, rising by 5.3 times. The net import of aquatic products decreased to 1.95 million tons, down by 57.5%.

Table 1-1　Net import of major foods in China from 1980 to 2021

Year	Net import (million tons)				
	Grain	Oil-bearing crops	Edible vegetable oils	Meats	Milk
1980	11.837	−0.115	0.183	−0.244	−0.029
1990	7.982	−0.648	2.064	−0.471	−0.228
2000	−1.023	2.308	2.044	−0.290	−0.401
2010	59.911	1.695	9.221	−0.037	3.499
2020	142.056	5.703	9.660	7.898	18.080
2021	162.650	5.532	10.270	7.308	21.950

Note: The data of net import in 2021 refer to the import and export data of major categories of grain in *China Agricultural Outlook Report (2022–2031)*. The data of net grain import in 2020 is the sum of all kinds of grain import and export data from customs. The net grain import in other years comes from the sum of four crops (cereals, potatoes, miscellaneous beans, and soybeans) in the food balance table of FAO.

1.1.3　Food supply has increased substantially, with sufficient quantity and abundant variety

From 1980 to 2021, the grain supply in China increased year by year, from 332.392 million tons to 822.802 million tons, with an increase of 1.5 times. In 2021, the supply of fruits and vegetables reached 300.822 million tons and 764.868 million tons respectively, increased by 46.0 times and 14.5 times from 1980. Edible vegetable oil increased to 38.82 million tons in 2021, with an increase of 10 times. The sugar supply increased to 19.955 million tons, which nearly doubled. The production of meats, eggs, milk and aquatic products reached 97.208 million tons, 33.988 million tons, 58.777 million tons and 66.587 million tons respectively, rising by 7.2 times, 11.0 times, 49.2 times and 14.0 times. With the greatly increased supply, food varieties are also increasing, and many kinds of fruits and seafood can be found in people's daily diets.

The per capita grain supply increased from 337.8 kg to 598.5 kg, reaching nearly 600 kg (Table 1-2). The self-sufficiency rate of grain increased from 95.9% in 1980 to 100.2% in 2000, and then decreased to 85.6% in 2021. The self-sufficiency rate of soybean decreased from 94.8% in 1980 to 14.5% in 2021. The self-sufficiency rate of meat decreased slightly from 102.2% in 1980 to 92.5% in 2021 (Figure 1-2). If all kinds of food were uniformly converted into energy, the energy self-sufficiency rate shows a downward trend, from 93.6% in 1980 to 80.2% in 2021 (Table 1-3).

Table 1-2   Per capita supply of main foods in China from 1980 to 2021

Year	Per capita supply (kg/year)					
	Grain	Edible oils	Vegetables	Fruits	Meats	Milk
1980	337.8	3.6	53.5	6.6	12.0	1.2
1990	389.7	6.9	109.6	15.7	24.1	3.8
2000	360.2	10.5	344.3	48.2	47.2	6.8
2010	455.2	21.0	412.5	145.9	58.8	24.9
2020	560.6	26.6	522.3	202.0	60.5	37.2
2021	598.5	27.5	541.5	213.0	68.8	41.6

Note: Grain includes cereals, potatoes (5 kg of fresh potatoes are equivalent to 1 kg of grain), miscellaneous beans and soybeans.

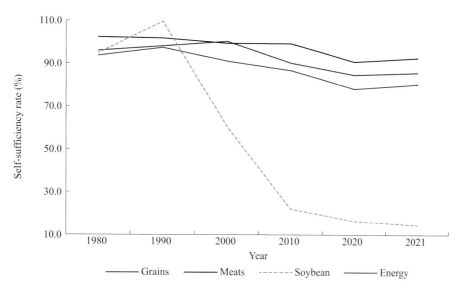

Figure 1-2   Self-sufficiency rate of main foods in China from 1980 to 2021

Table 1-3   Per capita energy production and supply in China from 1980 to 2021

Year	Self-sufficiency rate (%)	Domestic production (kcal/day)	Import (kcal/day)	Total supply (kcal/day)	Dietary supply (kcal/day)	Others (for industrial and feeding purposes) (kcal/day)
1980	93.6	2,314.6	157.5	2,472.1	2,146	326.1
1994	97.3	2,891.2	79.8	2,971.0	2,504	467.0
2000	90.9	3,019.8	302.2	3,322.0	2,808	514.0
2010	86.6	3,401.4	526.1	3,927.5	3,044	883.5
2020	78.0	3,599.4	1,013.5	4,612.9	3,445	1,167.9
2021	80.2	3,772.3	929.9	4,702.2	3,548	1,154.2

1.2   The consumption of animal products increased rapidly, and the consumption of food varieties was diversified

1.2.1   The consumption of rations decreased and then remains stable, and the consumption of miscellaneous grains decreased

The annual per capita consumption of rations (including cereals, potatoes, and miscellaneous beans; 5 kg of fresh potatoes are equivalent to 1 kg of grain) increased from 174.8 kg in 1980 to 202.9 kg in 1990, then declined slowly and gradually became stable, reaching 197.4 kg in 2021. The annual per capita consumption of cereals increased from 151.9 kg in 1980 to 187.0 kg in 1990, with an increase of 23.2%. After 1990, the consumption slowly decreased to 184.4 kg in 2021, with a decrease of 1.4%. Cereal consumption tends to be stable. However, from 1980 to 2021, the annual per capita consumption of potatoes and miscellaneous beans decreased from 89.5 kg and 5.0 kg to 59.1 kg and 1.2 kg respectively, with a decrease of 30.4% and 76.0%. It can be seen that the structure of ration consumption tends to be single, and it is necessary to take measures to promote the consumption of miscellaneous grains, to meet the daily nutrition and health needs of residents (Figure 1-3).

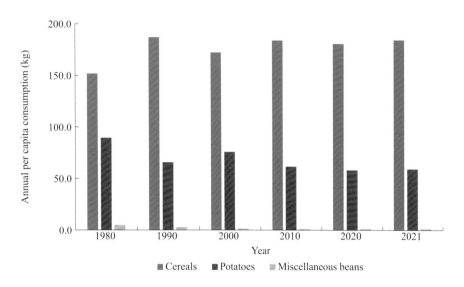

Figure 1-3   Consumption trends of cereals, potatoes and miscellaneous beans from 1980 to 2021

1.2.2   The consumption of animal products increased, which guaranteed the intake of high-quality protein

Since 1980, the consumption of animal products in China has shown a rapid growth tendency. The annual per capita consumption of meat increased from 12.0 kg in 1980 to 68.8 kg in 2021, with an increase of 56.8 kg. Among these, meat consumption increased by 2.9 times from 1980 to 2000, and then increased by 45.5% from 2000 to 2021. The annual per capita consumption of eggs increased from 2.5 kg in 1980 to 21.8 kg in 2021, with an increase of 19.3 kg. Before 2000, it increased by 5.2 times. After 2000, the tendency slowed down and increased by 41.6%. The annual per capita consumption of milk increased from 0.9 kg in 1980 to 37.0 kg in 2021, with an increase of 36.1 kg. From 1980 to 2000, it increased by 5.7 times. From 2000 to 2021, it increased by 5 times. The annual per capita consumption of aquatic products increased from 4.4 kg in 1980 to 39.5 kg in 2021, with an increase of 35.1 kg. From 1980 to 2000, it maintained a high-speed growth tendency, with an increase of 4.6 times. From 2000 to 2021, the growth slowed down, with an increase of 58.6%. Generally speaking, as a source of high-quality protein, the consumption of animal products greatly guarantees the nutrition and health needs of residents (Figure 1-4).

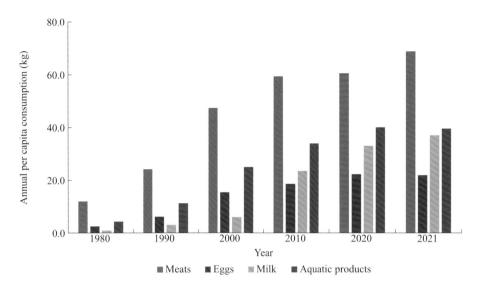

Figure 1-4   Consumption trends of animal products from 1980 to 2021

1.2.3   The consumption of fruits and vegetables continued to grow rapidly, which effectively ensures the intake of micronutrients

From 1980 to 2021, the annual per capita consumption of fruits increased from 5.9 kg to 180.0 kg, with an increase of 174.1 kg. From 1980 to 2000, the growth was rapid, with an increase of 6.0 times. From 2000 to 2021, although the growth rate declined, there was still an increase of 3.4 times. The annual per capita consumption of vegetables increased from 48.7 kg in 1980 to 463.5 kg in 2021, with an increase of 414.8 kg. From 1980 to 2000, it maintained a high-speed growth trend, with an increase of 5.2 times. From 2000 to 2021, the growth slowed down, with an increase of 52.8%. Fruits and vegetables are rich in dietary fiber, vitamins and minerals, which is important for guaranteeing the micronutrient intake of residents (Figure 1-5).

1.2.4   The consumption of vegetable oils increased obviously, while sugar consumption fluctuated steadily and increased slightly

The annual per capita consumption of vegetable oil increased year by year, from 3.0 kg in 1980 to 9.9 kg in 2021, with an increase of 6.9 kg. From 1980 to 2000, the growth rate was faster and doubled. From 2000 to 2021, the growth rate dropped to 62.3%, which remained at a high level. At present, the consumption of vegetable oils by residents has exceeded the upper limit of recommended intake. To prevent overweight and obesity caused by excessive intake of oils and fats, it is necessary to take corresponding measures to guide residents to appropriately reduce the consumption of fats including vegetable oil and other oils in the future (Figure 1-6).

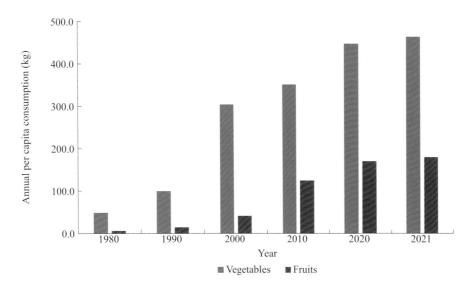

Figure 1-5　Consumption trends of vegetables and fruits from 1980 to 2021

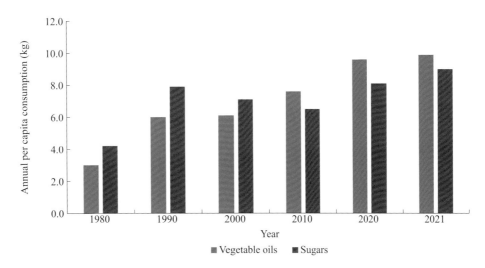

Figure 1-6　Consumption trends of vegetable oil and sugar from 1980 to 2021

The annual per capita consumption of sugar increased from 4.2 kg in 1980 to 9.0 kg in 2021, with an increase of 4.8 kg. From 1980 to 2000, the growth rate was faster, with an increase of 69.0%. From 2000 to 2021, the growth rate slowed down, with an increase of 26.8%. In the future, to avoid chronic diseases such as obesity caused by excessive sugar intake, residents should be guided to consume a moderate amount of sugar (Figure 1-6).

1.3   The nutrition of the resident has been greatly improved, and the supply of energy is sufficient

1.3.1   The energy, protein and fat supply of the resident continued to increase

The per capita daily energy supply of residents in China increased from 2,146.2 kcal in 1980 to 4,702.2 kcal in 2021, with an increase of 119.1%. In the same period, the daily protein and fat supply per capita increased from 53.4 g and 33.3 g to 102.8 g and 147.6 g, respectively, with an increase of 92.5% and 343.2% (Figure 1-7). The per capita fat supply in 2021 increased by more than 3 times compared with that of 1980, with the highest increase. At present, the per capita energy and protein supply are both higher than the recommended per capita daily intake target (2,200－2,300 kcal, 78 g) in 2020 put forward by the *China Food and Nutrition Development Program (2014－2020)*.

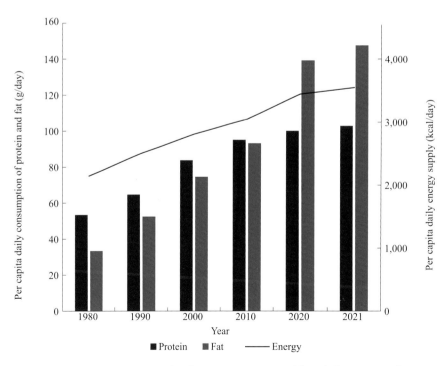

Figure 1-7   Per capita supply of energy, protein and fat of Chinese residents

The proportion of energy provided by carbohydrates decreased from 76.1% in 1980 to 51.0% in 2021, with a decrease of 25.1 percentage points. The proportion of energy provided by protein and fat increased from 10.0% and 14.0% in 1980 to 11.6% and 37.4% in 2021, with an increase of 1.6 percentage points and 23.4 percentage points, respectively (Table 1-4, Figure 1-8).

Table 1-4 Composition of nutrient sources for the energy supply of residents in China from 1980 to 2021

Year	Total energy		Carbohydrates		Proteins		Fats	
	Supply (kcal/day)	Percentage (%)	Supply (kcal/day)	Percentage (%)	Supply (kcal/day)	Percentage (%)	Supply (kcal/day)	Percentage (%)
1980	2,146.0	100.0	1,632.7	76.1	213.6	10.0	299.7	14.0
1990	2,504.0	100.0	1,774.0	70.8	258.4	10.3	471.6	18.8
2000	2,808.0	100.0	1,801.8	64.2	334.8	11.9	671.4	23.9
2010	3,045.0	100.0	1,827.1	60.0	380.0	12.5	837.9	27.5
2020	3,444.9	100.0	1,792.1	52.0	400.0	11.6	1,252.8	36.4
2021	3,547.8	100.0	1,808.2	51.0	411.2	11.6	1,328.4	37.4

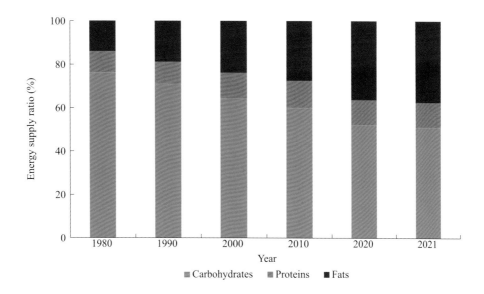

Figure 1-8 Composition of nutrient sources for the energy supply of residents in China from 1980 to 2021

1.3.2 The energy, protein and fat of animal food sources increased rapidly

The per capita daily supply of energy, protein and fat from plant food sources increased from 1981.0 kcal, 46.5 g and 18.5 g in 1980 to 2,821.2 kcal, 60.5 g and 90.2 g in 2021, with an increase of 42.4%, 30.1% and 387.6% respectively (Table 1-5).

The per capita daily supply of energy, protein and fat from animal food sources increased from 165.0 kcal, 6.9 g and 14.8 g in 1980 to 726.7 kcal, 42.3 g and 57.4 g in 2021, which increased by 3.4 times, 5.1 times and 2.9 times respectively. The increase in energy and fat supply from animal food sources may lead to the imbalance of the nutrition supply and increase the risk of nutrition-relevant chronic diseases.

From 1980 to 2021, the growth of daily energy supply per capita from plant food sources was higher than that from animal food sources, which were 840.2 kcal and 561.7 kcal respectively. However, the per capita daily supply of protein and fat from plant foods sources increased less than that from animal foods (Table 1-5). From 1980 to 2021, the proportions of energy, protein and fat provided by animal foods increased greatly, from 7.7%, 12.9% and 44.4% to 20.5%, 41.1% and 38.9%, respectively.

Table 1-5　Supply of energy, protein and fat from different food sources of residents in China from 1980 to 2021

Year	Food resources from the plant						Food resources from the animal					
	Energy		Protein		Fat		Energy		Protein		Fat	
	Supply (kcal/day)	Percentage (%)	Supply (g/day)	Percentage (%)	Supply (g/day)	Percentage (%)	Supply (kcal/day)	Percentage (%)	Supply (g/day)	Percentage (%)	Supply (g/day)	Percentage (%)
1980	1,981.0	92.3	46.5	87.1	18.5	55.6	165.0	7.7	6.9	12.9	14.8	44.4
1990	2,216.0	88.5	51.4	79.6	27.2	51.9	288.0	11.5	13.2	20.4	25.2	48.1
2000	2,290.0	81.6	56.5	67.5	31.3	42.0	518.0	18.4	27.2	32.5	43.4	58.2
2010	2,358.0	77.4	57.9	61.0	37.3	39.6	687.0	22.6	37.1	39.1	55.9	59.4
2020	2,786.0	80.9	60.8	60.8	87.5	62.9	658.9	19.1	39.2	39.2	51.6	37.1
2021	2,821.2	79.5	60.5	62.3	90.2	61.1	726.7	20.5	42.3	41.1	57.4	38.9

1.3.3　The energy, protein and fat supply of residents in China generally exceed the global average

At present, the per capita energy supply in China is lower than that of most developed countries in Europe and America, however, it is higher than that of developing countries such as India and South Africa. According to the production and supply level in 2019, the per capita daily energy supply in China was 3,347 kcal, which was lower than that of the United States, Germany, Canada, France and other countries (3,532 – 3,862 kcal), equivalent to that of Britain, Russia, Spain and other countries (3,348 – 3,395 kcal), and higher than that of South Africa, Japan and India (2,581 – 2,500 kcal). The per capita daily supply of protein in China was lower than that of Portugal and the United States (115.0 – 117.7 g), close to that of most developed countries (104.2 – 109.7 g), but higher than that of the Republic of Korea, Japan, South Africa and India (64.9 – 99.0 g). The per capita fat supply was also lower than most developed countries in Europe and America, but higher than some developing countries. The energy, protein and fat supplies of Chinese residents exceed the global average levels (Table 1-6).

Table 1-6　Per capita energy, protein and fat supply in different countries in 2019

Country	Energy (kcal/day)	Protein (g/day)	Fat (g/day)
America	3,862	115.0	180.1
Germany	3,559	104.2	149.6
Canada	3,539	108.6	156.0
France	3,532	109.7	151.5
Portugal	3,458	117.7	140.1
Republic of Korea	3,453	99.0	123.5
Australia	3,417	107.9	159.7
Britain	3,395	106.2	138.7
Russia	3,363	104.8	110.5
Spain	3,348	108.5	154.7
China	3,347	105.3	105.2

52

(Continued)

Country	Energy (kcal/day)	Protein (g/day)	Fat (g/day)
Brazil	3,246	93.8	131.4
Ukraine	3,036	90.1	91.6
South Africa	2,898	79.8	87.5
Japan	2,691	88.0	89.2
India	2,581	64.9	59.8
Average (Global)	2,963	83.2	88.0

2

Problems and challenges

2.1 Dietary imbalance, over-nutrition and nutrition deficiency coexist

2.1.1 The unhealthy lifestyle is still widespread

The research on global disease burden shows that an unreasonable diet is the main cause of disease incidence and mortality in China. The intakes of whole grains, dark vegetables, fruits, milk, fish, shrimp and soybeans are still lower than the recommended nutrient intakes. In China, only 20% of residents' intake of whole grains and miscellaneous grains can reach the recommended intake. Excessive intake of oil and salt is still widespread, and the consumption of sugary drinks is rising year by year. According to the *Scientific Research Report on Dietary Guidelines of Residents in China (2021)*, a considerable number of deaths of heart disease, stroke, and type 2 diabetes in China are related to dietary factors. In 2017, the number of deaths attributed to unreasonable diet was 3.1 million, which doubled as compared with 1.51 million in 2012. Among many factors of an unreasonable diet, high sodium intake had the greatest influence on cardiovascular metabolic death, accounting for 17.3% in 2012. The influence of high red meat intake on cardiovascular metabolic death had the fastest growth rate, in which the proportion increased by 1.5 times in recent 30 years. According to the study "Health effects of dietary risks in 195 countries, 1990–2017: a systematic analysis for the Global Burden of Disease Study 2017" published by *The Lancet*, a world-renowned medical journal, in 2019, in the list of deaths attributed to the diet structure, the top three risk factors were high-sodium diet, insufficient whole grain intake, and insufficient fruit intake (Figure 2-1).

2.1.2 The overweight and obesity among residents have become increasingly significant

From the perspective of the scientific dietary energy supply ratio, the upper limit

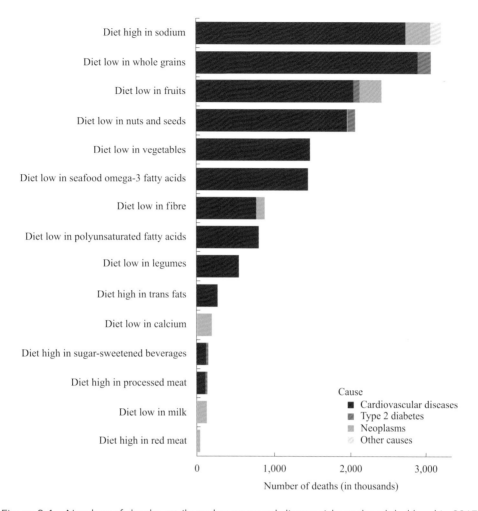

Figure 2-1　Number of deaths attributed to personal dietary risks at the global level in 2017

of the ratio of energy supply from fat is 30%. According to the *Report on Nutrition and Chronic Diseases of Residents in China (2020)*, the per capita ratio of energy supply from fat for both urban and rural residents exceeded the recommended upper limit. The ratio of energy supply from fat per standard person was 34.6%, that of urban and rural residents was 36.4% and 33.2% respectively, and that of rural residents exceeded 30% for the first time. In terms of the population, the proportion of people whose ratio of energy supply from fat exceeding 30.0% was 63.6%. The problem of overweight and obesity among residents had become increasingly significant, and the incidence of chronic diseases was still on the rise. At present, the overweight and obesity rate of the population aged 18 years and above in China was 50.7%, including an overweight rate of 34.3% and an obesity rate of 16.4%.

2.1.3　The micronutrient intake is still insufficient

In recent years, the intake of vitamin A, iron, zinc and other micronutrients in Chinese residents has improved. However, the resident's health status has still been affected by the hidden hunger problem. According to the *Report on Nutrition and Chronic Diseases of Residents in China (2020)*, the rate of low serum ferritin was 13.3% for residents aged 18 years and above, 11.2% for children and adolescents aged 6–17 years, and 54.4% for pregnant women. In 2018, the anemia rate of residents aged 18 years and above was still 8.7%, and that of pregnant women was even higher, reaching 13.6%. The rate of serum vitamin A deficiency was 4.7% for residents aged 18 years and above (including marginal deficiency rate, the same below), that of children and adolescents aged 6–17 years was 15.7%, and that of pregnant women was 9.6%.

2.2　Over-processing leads to a large loss of nutrition and a serious waste of food in the whole industry chain

2.2.1　Over-processing leads to more nutrition loss of staples

In our tradition, we have a habit of "seeking more essential food", and we are persistently pursuing "white, refined and beautiful" rice and flour. Thus, the flour becomes "snow pollen" and rice becomes "bright and refined". Almost all the epidermis and germ of the grain are removed from the polished rice and flour, leaving only the endosperm, resulting in a great loss of nutrients in grains. Previous research showed that, compared with whole wheat flour, the flour with higher processing degree lost 15% of protein, 83% of vitamin B_1, 67% of vitamin B_2, 50% of nicotinic acid, 80% of iron, 50% of calcium, 80% of zinc, etc. For rice, rice bran accounts for only 5%–8% of the mass of rice, while it concentrates 64% of the nutrients of rice. From the perspective of applications of by-products after processing, it is mainly used as feed raw materials, and a few of them are applied in the food processing industry. In China, the by-products after processing are fully utilized. Although the loss and waste seem to be small in quantity, the nutrition loss caused by excessive processing is relatively large. Consumption of over-processed rice and flour for a long period may lead to "hidden hunger" caused by the deficiency of nutrients including vitamins, minerals, etc., which has potential health risks.

2.2.2　The food loss is large in the front end of the industrial chain

According to the investigation by the Institute of Food and Nutrition Development of the Ministry of Agriculture and Rural Affairs, the overall food loss rate in China is 14.7%, slightly higher than the global average level (13.8%). From the perspective of the variety, the loss rates of vegetables, fruits, aquatic products, cereals, meats, milk and eggs are 25.9%, 13.1%, 8.1%, 7.0%, 6.6%, 4.6%, and 3.4% respectively. From the perspective of the link, the loss rates of agricultural production, post-production treatment, storage, processing and circulation are 4.3%, 4.9%, 2.6%, 0.5% and 2.3% respectively. The loss is mainly observed at the front end of the industrial chain. The loss from production and post-production treatment accounts for about 63% of the total loss. The loss from processing is the lowest, which is only 0.5% on average (Figure 2-2). According to the production data in 2021, the total food consumption in China is 300 million tons, which is equivalent to 164.7 trillion kcal of energy (9.5%), 7.1 million tons of protein (10.0%), and 2.53 million tons of fat (7.3%), respectively.

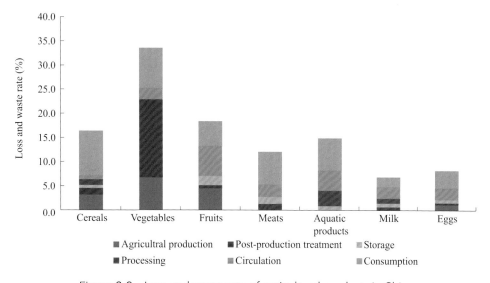

Figure 2-2　Loss and waste rate of agricultural products in China

(Data sources: Investigation by the animal food and nutrition policy team of the Institute of Food and Nutrition Development of the Ministry of Agriculture and Rural Affairs, the survey by Cheng Shengkui's team at the Institute of Geographical Sciences and Resources, Chinese Academy of Sciences)

2.2.3 Food waste is serious in the catering industry

According to the survey of typical cities by the Institute of Geographical Resources, Chinese Academy of Sciences, due to the "reputation-sensitive culture", food waste is common in cities. The per capita food waste is 93 g/meal (calculated as cooked food, the same as below), and the waste rate is 11.7%. The waste rate is even higher in business banquets and large-scale gatherings. In contrast, food waste in households is relatively limited, with a food waste rate of 4.8%. The weighted average food waste rate of households and restaurants is about 8.0%. According to the production data for 2021, the total amount of food waste in China is 160 million tons, which is equivalent to 146.4 trillion kcal of energy (8.4%), 5.69 million tons of protein (8.1%), and 2.41 million tons of fat (7.0%) respectively.

2.3 The concept of the scientific diet is lagging, and the population of food nutrition science needs to be strengthened

2.3.1 The cognitive transformation of food nutrition is relatively lagging, and many people still hold the concept of "eating-full and eating-well"

With the continuous development of the social economy in China, the diet and living standard of residents has improved day by day, and the dietary structure has changed greatly. However, the cognition of residents on food nutrition has not changed over time, and they still seek high-energy die and flavor experiences from previous ages short of food and clothing, without paying attention to the nutrition balance in their diet. According to the data from China Health and Nutrition Survey (CHNS), in 2015, women of childbearing age generally dominated food arrangements in Chinese families, whose nutritional knowledge level was 52%, and that of the elderly was as low as 30.5%. Even in Shanghai, where the nutritional knowledge level was higher than that of the whole country in the same period, in 2018, more than 50% of citizens still know nothing about the benefits of breastfeeding, and the same proportion of citizens don't know the health benefits of eating soybean food. More than half of middle-aged and elderly people don't pay attention to information such as production date, shelf life, nutritional composition table, and manufacturer when purchasing packaged food. Some wealthy people still regard fish and meat, oil and source, drinks and fast food, and foods with high salt and sugar content as the signs of "eating-well". With the rapid development of take-out and prefabricated foods, nutrition and health standards need to be improved. In 2021, the fast-food market reached 1,099.4 billion yuan, accounting for 23.4% of the catering industry in China. The proportions of eating out, ordering take-out, and purchasing prefabricated foods have gradually increased. There is still a lack of standardized guidance on nutrition, oil, salt and sugar in fast food.

2.3.2 The popularization guiding channels are chaotic, and the effective supply needs to be improved

The popularization of food and nutrition knowledge is not enough. First, limited attention has been paid to the popularization of food and nutrition. The funding is insufficient, the coverage rate of science popularization venues and bases is low, the incentive mechanism of science popularization practitioners is imperfect, and there is a shortage of talent. Second, the content of popularization is not targeted. The selected content deviates from the market demand. The real needs of consumers are often ignored or unrevealed. The content often focuses on simple science and technology, which is boring, lacking in pertinence, and far from actual living needs. Third, current popular science works are not systematic. It is lack of scientific, reasonable, professional, easy-to-understand, targeted, easy-to-operate and practical works. Most of the works are relatively simple in content and form, and their attraction and appeal need to be further improved.

2.3.3 Fewer young people can cook, so it is urgent to strengthen food education

At present, due to the finer division of labor and the increasing pressure of life, it is common that young people cannot cook. Apart from the reason for optimal time allocation, the most important reason is the lack of cultivation and training in cooking skills for students in the Chinese traditional education system. According to a scientific survey by ScienceNet.cn, nearly 60% of college students lack cooking skills. Coincidentally, an analysis report of Meituan takeout also indicated that the post-90s single people were the main consumers of ordering take-out, accounting for over 62%, and 40% of them could not cook. There is still much room for improving dietary cultivation in China, and consolidating healthy dietary skills.

2.3.4 The commercial orientation of food propaganda is obvious, and online celebrities dominate the communication mode

The popularization of food and nutrition is relatively less in regulatory authority organizations. However, food production, circulation and other business entities tend to carry out product marketing activities only considering their interests, target their products, and focus on consumers' needs and knowledge blind spots. These subjects conduct the subdivision and match according to the characteristics of channels, people and food categories. However, in terms of content, it garbles the context and selectively exaggerates the effect unilaterally. There are also some online platforms, especially the self-media, that claim to be "scientific experiments, pictures are the truth" while utilizing the online celebrities chased and worshipped by young people to conduct alarmist propaganda, create hot spots, mukbang, and sell goods, which mislead consumers, and damage the authority and credibility of formal food nutrition science guidance work.

2.4 The data on food resources are scarce, monitor and evaluation standards are lacking

2.4.1 The base data of food resources is unclear

General Secretary Xi Jinping proposes "Greater food", such as asking for food from forests, rivers, lakes, seas, and facility agriculture, expanding to wider biological resources, and seeking energy and protein from plants, animals, and microorganisms. But first of all, we are face with the problem of unclear base data. First, the data is unclear. At present, the data published by the National Bureau of Statistics only include macroscopic statistical data on major agricultural products. However, there is a lack of data on minor and special foods. The characteristics of resource stock, distribution, actual production capacity, and consumption structure of innovative, minor and special foods are unclear. Second, the degree and scope of development and utilization of food resources are unclear. Taking plant food resources as an example, in the China Botanical Subject Database jointly built by the Institute of Botany of Chinese Academy of Sciences and Kunming Institute of Botany of Chinese Academy of Sciences, more than 155,000 items of plant data are collected, of which less than 1,200 items are recorded in the database of edible plants. In 2021, China Useful Plant Resources Database published by Zhuang Huifu et al. extracted 51,949 records of useful plants in China from all kinds of local chronicles and literature, including 5,247 records of edible plants (The data contains duplicate records, including plants used for condiments, foods and drinks that need to be processed). This set of data is the database with relatively comprehensive records of current edible plant resources. However, this set of data only records the names (Chinese and Latin), application descriptions, and classifications of edible plant resources, without sorting out the development and utilization degree and application scope of these food resources. It is not sufficient to provide basic data support for the country to adjust the strategic layout of food resources development and utilization in the future. Third, the characteristics of nutrition are unclear. The nutrition characteristics of food provide basic support for formulating nutrition policies and solving malnutrition problems, such as obesity and hidden hunger. China has paid attention to quantity safety and quality safety for the long term, while the attention to nutrition safety has just started. There are only a limited variety of foods in the existing Food Composition Table, which only contains conventional macro and micronutrients, while the data on functional nutrients, flavor substances, and active factors are missing. In addition, the existing *Food Composition Table* lacks a regular updating mechanism, and the data update is slow. Thus, it can neither provide important support for the adjustment of nutrition policy or agricultural policy.

2.4.2 There is no standard for monitoring and evaluating the nutritional quality of food resources

First, the quality monitoring system is not perfect. The existing monitoring system focuses on safety and health indicators such as agricultural and veterinary drug residues, heavy metals, biotoxins and microorganisms. However, the evaluation of nutrition quality is ignored. Second, food nutrition evaluation is still in the initial stage. The existing evaluation indicators are not perfect, the evaluation methods are not standardized, the grading standards are lacking, and it is difficult to effectively regulate the market. Thus, many food resources are still difficult to get out of forests, grasslands, marine lakes, and remote areas. Third, there is no regular monitoring mechanism or system. In terms of resource distribution, China has a vast land area and rich agricultural food resources, and some food resources are located in remote areas, mountainous areas, and ethnic minority areas. The types, quantities and nutrition characteristics are very complex. At present, the situation is still confusing. In terms of administration, it involves different departments such as the Ministry of Agriculture and Rural Affairs, the Ministry of Natural Resources, the National Health and Health Commission, and the State Administration of Market Supervision, etc. However, no regular monitoring mechanism has been established, and there is also a lack of corresponding laws and regulations.

2.4.3　The research investment in food resources is insufficient, and scientific and technological innovation ability is weak

Food is closely related to the national economy and public health. However, at present, the scientific research investment in food resource monitoring and evaluation has been insufficient in China. In addition, the investment has been mainly concentrated in the production of important agricultural products such as grain. Currently, the investment in agricultural science and technology development accounts for only about 0.7%, which is far behind the investment intensity of more than 2% in developed countries. In addition to traditional agricultural and livestock products, the investment in the development and utilization of special foods is more limited. Affected by insufficient investment in science and technology, the construction of talent teams, discipline systems, and platform conditions lag behind, which seriously restricts the improvement of innovation ability.

3

**Transition to
nutrition and health**

3.1 Developing nutrition-oriented agriculture, and accelerating the transformation of the food system

Developing nutrition-oriented agriculture is an important measure to promote the nutritional transformation of the food system, support the optimization of residents' dietary structure, and eliminate malnutrition. We should take sustainable development as the goal, nutrition orientation as the concept, and resources as the starting point, thus reconstructing the agricultural industrial chain and food value chain.

3.1.1 Accelerating the formulating of nutrition standards for agricultural products, guiding the technological innovation of animal and plant breeding and planting, and promoting the construction of a nutrition-oriented food production system

There are severe challenges in food production including an insufficient supply of high-quality products and an obvious decline in micronutrients. It is urgent to change the concept from "production-oriented" to "paying equal attention to production and nutrition". First, it is necessary to accelerate and promote the formulation of a nutrition standard system for agricultural products, giving priority to formulating several demonstration standards with mature technology and urgent industrial needs. Associations, enterprises, and other parties should be guided to actively participate in the standard construction, and promote the transformation of food production to be nutrient-oriented. Second, nutritional quality should be considered an important goal of breeding and production. The construction of a comprehensive quality evaluation system should be accelerated, including nutritional quality, sensory quality, processing quality, etc. More new varieties of animals and plants with high nutritional density and quality should be cultivated. Third, the research and development of nutrition-oriented new technologies for planting and breeding should be promoted, thus producing more high-quality agricultural products with specific nutritional functions.

3.1.2 Encouraging moderate processing and precise processing, promoting agricultural product processing to reduce losses and increase efficiency, and accelerating the construction of a nutrition-oriented food processing system

At present, over-pursuit of flavor and taste leads to excessive nutrition loss. Because of this problem, it is urgent to innovate the concept, adhere to the guiding ideology of "giving priority to nutrition and health, and giving consideration to flavor and taste", and promote moderate processing, precise processing and flexible manufacturing. First, the rule of nutrition quality changing in the whole industrial chain of agricultural products should be systematically explored. It can provide theoretical support for technological innovation of moderate and precise processing. Second, the level of primary processing and commercialization in the place of origin should be improved, thus avoiding over-processing. Enterprises should be guided to reasonably determine the processing degree of rations such as wheat and rice. Innovative health products should be developed, such as special flour, whole wheat flour, special rice and brown rice. Third, wheat bran, rice bran, peel and pomace should be taken full advantage of to develop vegetable oils, dietary fibers, protein products and other products, thus improving the comprehensive utilization efficiency of food.

3.1.3 Incorporating nutrition orientation into all policies, increasing the affordability and accessibility of healthy meals, and accelerating the construction of a nutrition-oriented consumption system

Because of the unreasonable dietary structure and unscientific dietary concept of residents, it is urgent to optimize and improve the policy system for guiding consumption. First, the existing nutrition labeling system should be improved, the nutrition labeling system of prepackaged foods should be changed and transformed, the Front-of-package (FOP) labels and nutrition labeling system of fresh agricultural products should be vigorously promoted. Second, efforts should be made to improve the food consumption environment and create a nutritious and healthy canteen. For foods containing high contents of salt, oil and sugar, restriction policies should be explored such as food labeling or taxation. Third, the nutrition content should be defined in social protection policies. For the food aid of vulnerable groups, such as nutrition improvement plans for students in rural compulsory education, high nutrition quality, and balanced collocation should be ensured, as well as enhancing the affordability and availability of a healthy diet.

3.2 Developing the third ration, and improving the diversity of staples

Abundant food variety is the cornerstone to ensure a balanced diet for residents. The food and Agriculture Organization of the United Nations (FAO) regards biodiversity as the fundamental guarantee of food security and nutrition. The traditional concept of "five kinds of cereal are for the raising" has always been an important content of Chinese food culture. According to the monitoring data on the nutrition and health status of residents in China from 2015 to 2017, the intake of miscellaneous grains and potatoes accounted for only 17.9% of the total intake of grains and potatoes. The ration variety is too concentrated, and the intake of miscellaneous grains and whole grains is insufficient, which not only reduces the diversity of staples thus bringing huge health risks, but also leads to great pressure on food security. Miscellaneous grains and whole grains are the best choices to optimize the ration structure and balance dietary nutrition. There are many varieties of miscellaneous grains, most of which do not compete for water and land with staples. In addition, they are rich in B vitamins, dietary fiber and micronutrients, which are important varieties to optimize the ration structure and improve the nutrition supply, presenting obvious nutrition advantages and irreplaceability. Compared with wheat and rice, the marginal effect of developing coarse cereals is higher, and there will be obvious results after making efforts. It is urgent and imperative to guide the consumption of miscellaneous grains. We should educate the consumers to scientifically understand the role of miscellaneous grains in achieving a healthy diet and balanced nutrition, cultivate consumption habits, increase the ratio of miscellaneous grains as staples, and promote the return of miscellaneous grains to the dominant position. Through continuous effects, the third ration can be developed. We should strive to double the intake of miscellaneous grains and potatoes to 35% by 2035.

3.2.1   Optimizing the regional layout of coarse cereals, building an industrial chain that meets the nutritional and health needs of residents, and promoting the industrial quality and efficiency

First, optimizing the production layout of miscellaneous grains. According to the guiding principle of the national *Outline of the Construction Plan of Advantage Areas of Characteristic Agricultural Products*, the planting of miscellaneous grains, miscellaneous beans, and potatoes can be actively developed in Loess Plateau, Inner Mongolia and the area along the Great Wall, Northeast area, Northwest wind-blown arid area, Taihang Mountain area and Southwest rocky desertification area. Second, developing the miscellaneous grains processing industry, improving the upstream and downstream industrial chain. The standardized and large-scale production of traditional miscellaneous grains should be improved, then promoting "primary production" and "tertiary production" through "secondary production". The system innovations of the industrial chain should be explored and promoted, such as the "Chain director system". The docking platform can be established, covering breeding and extension experts, production, processing, trading, circulation and retail enterprises, thus achieving a deep connection between the innovation chain and the industrial chain. Third, improving the planting efficiency and encouraging miscellaneous grains production. The mechanism for realizing high quality and high prices in the miscellaneous grains industry should be explored. Then, traditional miscellaneous grains production should be promoted to jump out from the main production areas to the national market, promote consumption, and then improve the planting effectiveness of farmers.

3.2.2   Promoting the breeding of new varieties of miscellaneous grains and the innovation of high quality, high yield and high-efficiency technology, and improving the supply of high-quality raw materials

First, promoting the breeding and extension of new varieties of coarse cereals.

Guided by market demand, the nutritional quality, processing quality, and palatability of existing varieties are scientifically evaluated, thus screening the varieties with high quality and good palatability. The "breeding, cultivating and expanding" system of miscellaneous grain seeds should be established, focusing on "who will cultivate, who will breed, who will supply and who will expand". The industry development of miscellaneous grain seeds should be vigorously promoted. Second, accelerating the innovation of high-quality, high-yield and high-efficiency production technology. We should strengthen the technological innovation for quality control, equipment creation of simple and light specialized agricultural machinery, the combination of improved seeds and technologies, as well as the technical integration modes, and production specifications of agricultural machinery and technology integration. It aims to improve production efficiency and quality, and increase the supply of high-quality raw materials.

3.2.3 Breaking through the key technologies of miscellaneous grains production and processing as soon as possible, and improving the flavor and taste

Miscellaneous grain products are difficult to cook, rough in taste, and hard to digest and absorb, which are important factors for restricting consumption. First, developing modern food processing technologies such as micronization, low-temperature baking, and microwave curing for improving taste and cooking characteristics. It aims to realize the maintenance and efficient utilization of active ingredients such as phenols, polysaccharides, lipids and phytosterols in miscellaneous grains, and achieve the best balance among processing accuracy, edible quality and activity maintenance. Second, guiding the enterprises to customize scientific nutrition matching according to the dietary and nutritional needs of different groups of people, and to develop miscellaneous grain products and whole-grain foods, such as fast-cooked miscellaneous grain products, ready-to-eat meal replacement powder, etc. It aims to realize the deep integration of taste, nutrition and health.

3.3 Implementing a white meat growth plan, and promoting a healthy low-carbon diet

White meat, represented by poultry meat and aquatic products, has the characteristics of low content of fat and high content of unsaturated fatty acid. It is the first choice of healthy and high-quality protein sources, which is increasingly favored by consumers. In 2016, global poultry production has surpassed pork, becoming the largest meat product in the world. In 1990, in the United States, poultry production surpassed beef, accounting for 37.6% of total meat production, making it the most-consumed meat product. In 2019, poultry production in the United States accounted for 47.5%. The main reason for the rapid growth of poultry production is the high feed conversion rate, which is superior to red meat products such as beef, mutton and pork. Thus, the pressure on resources and the environment is significantly less than on other meat products. In addition, the increase in white meat intake can effectively reduce fat intake. According to the weighted calculation of data from the *China Food Composition Table*, the fat is 9.4 g in every 100 g of poultry meat, which is 20.7 g lower than that of pork. It is preliminarily predicted that the meat consumption of residents in China will reach a peak of 75 kg in 2035. Under the condition that other meat products remain unchanged, the increase in meat consumption is partly supplemented by poultry or aquatic products. Under the development goal of "carbon neutrality and peak carbon dioxide emissions", it is of great significance to consider the factors such as nutrition and health of residents, not exerting excessive pressure on resources and the environment. Thus, it is suggested to implement the strategy of "promoting white meat".

3.3.1 Formulating policies to promote the development of poultry and aquatic products

The development of poultry and aquatic products should be further promoted in livestock breeding, and be treated as a strategic industry that should be given priority to development in the agricultural industry. Support for breeding, slaughtering and processing, and environmental treatment should be provided. Development-oriented and policy-oriented financial institutions should be guided to increase their support for the poultry industry. In particular, we should make full use of agriculture-supported, small and re-lending-supported, and subsidized loan policies, thus supporting enterprises to develop production.

3.3.2 Strengthening critical technology innovation in the breeding of poultry and aquatic variety

In the national science and technology plan, we should enhance the support for poultry and aquatic breeding, focus on variety breeding and expanding, support the establishment of a national breeding base, guide breeding enterprises to establish a close benefit linkage mechanism with large-scale propagation farms/ponds, enhance the variety development and transformation capabilities of poultry and aquatic products.

3.3.3 Promoting the scale, standardization, and intelligence of industry development

We should take the construction of high-standard farms/ponds as the starting point, improve the construction of biological safety systems during the production of poultry meat and aquatic products, improve the utilization level of intelligent facilities and equipment, upgrade the modern breeding level of poultry and aquatic products, and promote the sustainable and healthy development of the industry. The popular science propaganda for the safe and healthy breeding of white meat should be strengthened, and consumers' trust in the quality of white meat products and the concept of consuming healthy animal food should be established.

3.4 Reducing losses depending on science and technology, practicing saves and eliminating waste

China has a large-scale agriculture and population, while the water and soil resources are limited. So, it is increasingly difficult to increase food production.

Reducing food loss and waste is particularly important for ensuring food security and sustainable development of the food system in China. The rate of food loss and waste in China can be 22.7%. It is estimated that about half of the loss (11.35 percentage points) can be saved, equal to 230 million tons of food, which can be converted into 155.7 trillion kcal of heat. It can meet the nutritional needs of 190 million people for one year, reduce the use of 250 million mu of cultivated land resources, 150 million cubic meters of water resources consumption, and 160 million tons of greenhouse gas emissions.

3.4.1   Increasing the investment, strengthening the infrastructure and technology support for reducing food losses and wastes

We should improve the mechanization and intelligence level of harvesting, storage, segmentation and other links, promote the application of advanced cold-chain equipment, increase the proportion of cold storage and fresh-keeping processing in production areas, and accelerate the completion of the "first mile" short board in cold-chain production areas of agricultural products, promote the development of standards in key links and key areas for reducing food losses and wastes, and promote the timely application of advanced technologies, processes, equipment, etc. in food loss reduction practices.

3.4.2   Shortening food transporting mileage, and reducing circulation loss of fresh agricultural products

With agricultural production gradually concentrated in the advantageous producing areas, the phenomenon of "southern vegetables and fruits being transported to the north" has become increasingly prominent. The circulation links and long distances cause a large amount of food losses. Encouraging the application of suburban agricultural land in large and medium-sized cities, intensifying the construction of bases for fresh agricultural products that are not resistant to storage and transportation, such as vegetables, and ensuring that the self-sufficiency rate is at least above 30%. The coordination between the main production areas and key regions of important cities should be strengthened, the distribution radius should be rationally set, thus improving the circulation efficiency of agricultural products, shortening the food transporting mileage, and improving the efficiency and resilience of the food supply system.

3.4.3 Applying multiple measures, and vigorously opposing food losses and wastes

The implementation of the *Anti-food Waste Law of the People's Republic of China* should be accelerated, further refining supporting regulations, formulating and improving relevant supporting regulations as soon as possible, and establishing a long-term mechanism to oppose food waste. Restraining the food waste in the catering industry, encouraging "individual serving" and "small proportion meals", and supporting catering enterprises to charge appropriate fees for limiting the waste behaviors of consumers. Enhancing the publicity and education of anti-food waste, actively advocating the civilized, healthy and scientific food culture, improving the awareness of the anti-food waste of the whole society, and creating a social awareness of "saving is glorious and waste is shameful".

3.5 Starting from children and person who cooks, and promoting healthy diet education

Healthy diet education is not only related to individual health but also related to the inheritance of national diet culture and the sustainable development of human groups. Healthy diet education is a systematic project. The "campus" and "family" are two critical links.

3.5.1 Promoting food education in the campus, and incorporating food education into the teaching system of kindergartens, primary and secondary schools

Food education is the premise and foundation of intellectual education, and it is the first selected strategy to improve the nutrition level of children, adolescents, and even the whole society. Food education should be put in the same important position as "moral, intellectual, physical, aesthetics, and labor education", and incorporating food education into the teaching system of kindergartens, primary and secondary schools. Dietary knowledge and good dietary habits should be systematically incorporated into preschool education. In addition, food can be applied as the carrier to guide and cultivate the consciousness of morality, culture, nutrition science and sustainable development. It is necessary to promote the compilation of food education textbooks and teacher training in primary and secondary schools, focus on improving teachers' knowledge and cultivation of food nutrition, and give full play to the dominant position and enthusiasm of teachers in food education. The full-time dietitians should be set in kindergartens, primary and secondary school canteens, preparing nutritious meals in line with the growth and development stages of students, giving full play to the exemplary roles of student canteens in nutrition education, thus improving food nutrition cultivation of students.

3.5.2　Promoting the food education in the family, and playing the leading roles of the person who cooks in food education

Food education in the family has the advantages of multiple measures, low cost and wide coverage, which has been used by the government, health departments, and nutrition circles of many countries as the main measures to improve the nutrition status of children, adolescents and families. We should actively promote food education in the family, advocate eating at home, conduct food education classes for the person who cooks, and improve food nutrition knowledge and skills. Food nutrition research institutions and social organizations at all levels should actively conduct the investigation, communication, guidance and practice on the models related to food conditions in the family. Slow food in the family should be actively advocated while standardizing the development of fast food.

3.5.3　Strengthening the training of mainstream science popularization teams, and promoting the reconstruction of communication pattern

Governments at all levels should fully understand the significance of nutrition science popularization to the construction of "Healthy China", take nutrition science popularization as an important strategic measure, and increase investment. Mainstream media, food nutrition-relevant research institutes at all levels, colleges and universities, societies associations, and etc. should actively take responsibility for food nutrition science popularization, create an innovative mode of communication, and play their roles as main channels and leaders in food nutrition science popularization. The food and nutrition science popularization reward system should be gradually improved, researchers and employees in the field of food nutrition should be encouraged to actively engage in science popularization. Authoritative food nutrition think tanks, such as the National Food and Nutrition Advisory Committee, should further improve the construction of relevant new media platforms, and intensify the construction of popular science propaganda and practice bases. The science popularization industry should strengthen self-discipline and supervision, and relevant departments should increase the punishment of rumors.

3.6 Conducting a general survey of food resources, and building a food monitoring and evaluation system

According to the requirements of the "Greater food" concept, at present, the monitoring and evaluation of food nutrition quality in China still lack scientific standards, and the construction of scientific and technological conditions lags, making it difficult to support the efficient development and utilization of food resources. Therefore, it is necessary to establish a database of food resources and their nutrition characteristics, as well as a monitoring and evaluation system.

3.6.1 Conducting monitoring of food resources

The food monitoring system covering all regions and categories should be established, and the monitoring indicators and methods should be standardized. The database for the development and utilization of food resources and the database for food nutrition and quality monitoring should be established by applying multi-source and multi-modal data fusion cognitive computing technology, basic agricultural product standard knowledge graphs, database technology, multi-source meteorological data technology, block-chain technology, remote sensing technology, electronic fence identification technology, etc. by fully integrating the existing food data resources from various departments.

3.6.2 Performing the quality evaluation of characteristic food resources

Focusing on the nutritional components, sensory characteristics, and active factors of food resources, protein omics, metabolomics, and food omics techniques can be applied to perform the high-throughput screen and identification of the characteristics of food resources. The multi-dimensional evaluation method based on the characteristics of production areas should be established. Identifying food resources of different production areas, varieties and qualities, developing geographical indication products, and formulating grading standards, thus accurately exerting the unique functions, nutrition and health values of different food resources.

3.6.3 Promoting fundamental research, technological innovation, and demonstration utilization of food resources

Building national key laboratories for food resource monitoring and nutrition evaluation, strengthening the construction of a food resource innovation platform, and establishing a discipline system and talent training system for food resource evaluation. The demonstration and development of the food resources industry should be promoted, such as building industrial demonstration bases, strengthening information demonstration, and utilizing big data, artificial intelligence and cloud computing, thus providing important technological support for increasing food diversity, nutrition diversity and ecological diversity.

References

艾媒数据中心，2022. 餐饮行业数据分析：中国男性网民食用中式快餐频率与女性不同［EB/OL］. 艾媒网. https://www.iimedia.cn/c1061/84785.html.

餐饮新纪元，2020. 90后单身人群是点外卖的主力军占比超62%，其中40%的人不会做饭［EB/OL］.［2021-09-12］. https://www.163.com/dy/article/FGD8OHUK0519DCKC.html.

陈萌山，2021. 发展营养导向型农业建设健康中国［J］. 农村工作通讯（7）：21-23.

陈思佳，沈欣，郭若宜，等，2020. 亲子健康饮食教育模式对学龄前儿童早餐质量的影响［J］. 中国学校卫生，41（5）：769-771.

程蓓，2019. 食育的中国之策——基于日美两国的经验［J］. 中国德育（4）：14-18.

樊晓莉，孙桂菊，2022. 中国育龄女性膳食营养知识水平变化趋势及影响因素分析［J］. 中国公共卫生，38（6）：787-791.

顾锦春，范含信，2022. 乡村振兴背景下加强农村中学健康饮食教育的思考［J］. 现代农村科技（9）：93-95.

国家发展和改革委员会，农业农村部，国家林业和草原局，2022. 特色农产品优势区建设规划纲要［EB/OL］.［2022-09-12］. http://www.gov.cn/xinwen/2017-10/31/content_5235803.htm.

国家统计局，2021. 2021中国统计年鉴［M］. 北京：中国统计出版社.

国家卫生健康委疾病预防控制局，2021. 中国居民营养与慢性病状况报告（2020年）［M］. 北京：人民卫生出版社.

韩凤芹，周孝，史卫，等，2018. 我国财政科普投入及其效果评价［J］. 财政科学，36（12）：19-36.

黄家章，卢士军，姚远，等，2020. 基于文献计量的国际营养导向型农业研究进展可视化分析［J］. 中国农业科技导报，22（9）：11-21.

金妍，2022. 新媒体视野下科普传播模式及发展策略［J］. 中国报业（2）：90-91.

联合国粮食及农业组织，2019. 营养导向型农业与食物系统：干预措施［M］. 孙君茂，黄家章，卢士军，译. 北京：中国农业科学技术出版社.

卢士军，黄家章，吴鸣，等，2019. 营养导向型农业的概念、发展与启示［J］. 中国农业科学，52（18）：3083-3088.

马冠生，张曼，2019. 儿童饮食行为调查：经常吃快餐、喝饮料危害儿童健康［EB/OL］.［2021-09-12］. https://zhuanlan.zhihu.com/p/82106526.

农业农村部市场预警专家委员会，2020. 中国农业展望报告2020—2029［M］. 北京：中国农业科学技术出版社.

农业农村部市场预警专家委员会，2021. 中国农业展望报告2021—2030［M］. 北京：中国农业科学技术出版社.

农业农村部市场预警专家委员会，2022. 中国农业展望报告2022—2031［M］. 北京：中国农业科学技术出版社.

孙君茂，卢士军，江晓波，等，2019. 营养导向型农业国内外政策规划与启示［J］. 中国农业科学，52（18）：3089-3096.

唐洪涛，夏蕊，孙学安，等，2020. 家庭教育的重要一环：食育［J］. 中国校外教育（8）：1-2.

唐闻佳，2019. 超半数市民不知母乳喂养能让婴儿少生病，上海首发"健康素养72条"补常识短板［EB/OL］. ［2021-09-12］. https://wenhui.whb.cn/third/baidu/201903/27/252 246.html.

王文月，臧明伍，张辉，等，2022. 我国食品科技创新力量布局现状与发展建议［J］. 食品科学，43（13）：336-341.

王瑜，黄程佳，2016. 我国幼儿食育必要性及其促进策略［J］. 学前理论教育，32（4）：15-19.

杨舒，2022. 新时代推进科普工作系统布局已形成——专家解读《关于新时代进一步加强科学技术普及工作的意见》［N/OL］. 光明日报. ［2021-09-12］. https://share.gmw.cn/news/2022-09/06/content_36004950.htm.

中共中央办公厅，2022. 关于新时期进一步加强科学技术普及工作的意见［EB/OL］. ［2022-09-12］. https://www.ncsti.gov.cn/zcfg/zcwj/202209/t20220905_96313.html.

中国疾病预防控制中心营养与健康所，2019. 中国食物成分表：标准版［M］. 6版. 北京：北京大学医学出版社.

中国营养学会，2022. 中国居民膳食指南［M］. 北京：人民卫生出版社.

中研普华研究院，2021. 2022—2027年版快餐产品入市调查研究报告［EB/OL］. ［2021-09-12］https://3g.163.com/dy/article/HCN7MHDR0518H9Q1.html.

诸葛卫东，张一婧，傅一程，2020. 由奖励制度看日本科普策略与实践的发展方向［J］. 自然辩证法通讯，42（11）：101-110.

庄会富，王亚楠，王趁，等，2021. 中国有用植物资源数据库［J/OL］. 中国科学数据. ［2021-09-12］. DOI: 10.11922/csdata.2021.0006.zh.

GBD 2017 Diet Collaborators，2019. Health effects of dietary risks in 195 countries，1990—2017: A systematic analysis for the Global Burden of Disease Study 2017［J］. The Lancet，393（10184）：1958-1972.

KIRK D，CATAL C，TEKINERDOGAN B，2021. Precision nutrition: A systematic literature review［J］. Computers in Biology and Medicine，133: 104365.

XUE L，LIU X，LU S，et al.，2021. China's food loss and waste embodies increasing environmental impacts［J］. Nature Food，2（7）：519-528.

Appendix I Production of various foods in China from 1980 to 2021

Production of various foods in China from 1980 to 2021

Year	Grain	Cereals	Potatoes	Miscellaneous beans	Vegetables	Fruits	Meats	Milks	Eggs	Aquatic products	Soybean	Nut	Sugars	Oils
1980	320,555	277,190	158,700	6,700*	53,160*	6,793	12,054	1,141	2,800*	4,497	7,940	3,600	3,494	3,317*
1985	379,108	337,072	143,625	5,500*	92,775*	11,639	19,265	2,499	5,347	7,052	10,500	6,664	7,256	5,240*
1990	446,243	401,690	130,180	6,120*	129,101*	18,744	28,570	4,157	7,946	14,273	11,000	6,368	8,657	5,922*
1995	466,618	416,116	137,165	4,373	257,267	42,146	52,601	5,764	16,767	29,530	13,502	10,235	9,528	7,788*
2000	462,175	405,224	163,130	4,691	444,679	62,261	60,139	8,274	21,820	37,062	15,409	14,437	9,162	11,356*
2005	484,022	427,760	184,260	5,229	564,515	161,201	69,389	27,534	24,381	44,199	16,348	14,342	11,342	15,700*
2006	498,042	450,992	173,425	4,955	539,531	17,102	70,999	29,446	24,240	45,836	15,082	12,887	12,552	16,244*
2007	504,139	459,630	135,065	4,298	575,378	176,594	69,164	29,471	25,467	47,475	12,793	13,815	14,499	15,911*
2008	534,343	485,694	137,090	4,510	586,692	182,791	73,709	30,106	26,996	48,956	15,709	14,635	15,607	16,750*
2009	539,409	492,433	142,150	3,822	591,395	190,937	77,067	29,951	27,519	51,164	15,224	14,604	14,096	18,383*
2010	559,113	511,967	139,645	3,308	572,649	200,954	79,936	30,389	27,769	53,730	15,410	15,136	13,564	19,288*

(Continued)

Year	Grain	Cereals	Potatoes	Miscellaneous beans	Vegetables	Fruits	Meats	Milks	Eggs	Aquatic products	Soybean	Nut	Sugars	Oils
2011	588,493	540,617	142,135	3,755	597,666	210,186	80,230	31,099	28,304	56,032	14,879	15,302	13,996	19,992*
2012	612,226	566,590	146,215	3,370	616,245	220,915	84,711	31,749	28,854	55,021	13,436	15,792	14,942	21,183*
2013	630,482	586,504	144,150	3,017	631,980	227,481	86,328	30,008	29,055	57,442	12,407	16,109	15,066	21,039*
2014	639,648	596,015	142,770	3,959	649,487	233,026	88,179	31,599	29,303	60,019	12,686	15,901	14,506	22,613*
2015	660,603	618,184	139,940	2,758	664,251	245,246	87,495	31,798	30,461	62,110	12,367	15,961	13,458	23,920*
2016	660,435	616,666	136,465	2,912	674,342	244,052	86,283	30,640	31,605	63,795	13,596	16,361	13,411	22,899*
2017	661,607	616,205	136,315	3,134	691,927	252,419	86,544	30,386	30,963	64,453	15,283	17,092	13,655	24,137*
2018	657,892	610,036	139,930	3,236	703,467	256,884	86,246	30,746	31,283	64,577	15,967	17,332	14,325	24,664*
2019	663,843	613,697	143,270	3,227	721,026	274,008	77,588	32,012	33,090	64,804	18,092	17,520	14,603	24,910**
2020	669,492	616,743	144,135	3,273	749,129	286,924	77,484	34,401	34,678	65,490	19,602	17,993	14,417	27,870**
2021	682,848	632,757	149,370	3,255**	775,488	299,702	89,900	36,827	34,088	64,637	16,400**	18,308	13,745	28,550**

Data source: *China Statistical Yearbook 1981 – 2021*, in which standard * data is from FAO food balance sheet, and standard ** data is from *China Agriculture Outlook Report.*

Appendix Ⅱ Events of food and nutrition at home and abroad in 2021

In 2021, the COVID-19 epidemic swept the world, which made significant effects on global health. Because of this situation, the international community has taken measures to improve the nutritional status. The transformation of the food system has been advocated to meet the needs of sustainable development and health, and to realize "zero hunger" worldwide. In China, people in the food nutrition field mainly focus on food security, food waste reduction, food system and food nutrition development program, etc. This reflects that when food quantity safety is basically guaranteed in China, with the improvement of residents' living standards and the upgrading of consumption structure, food quality safety has become a realistic high-level demand of food safety strategy. In this part, the typical representative events are mainly reviewed.

On January 4th, the Fifth Plenary Session of the 19th the Communist Party of China (CPC) Central Committee deliberated and approved *Central Committee of the Communist Party of China's Proposal on Formulating the 14th Five-Year Plan for National Economic and Social Development and the Long-term Goals for 2035*. In the No.1 Central Document of 2021, the issue of food security was placed in a prominent position. It is proposed to firmly hold the two bottom lines: ensuring national food security and not returning to poverty on a large scale. To promote the steady and healthy development of the economy and society, we must focus on the major strategic needs of the country, stabilize the basic agricultural situation, give importance to "agriculture, farmer and rural area" issues, and continue to comprehensively promote rural revitalization. In 2021, the structural reform on the supply side of agriculture was further advanced. The sown area of grain has remained stable, the output has reached more than 0.65 trillion kg. The pig industry has developed steadily. The quality of agricultural products and the level of food safety have been further improved. The farmers' income continued to grow faster than that of urban residents, and the achievements in tackling poverty have been continuously consolidated.

On January 12th, World Health Organization released the *Action framework for developing and implementing public food procurement and service policies for a healthy diet*. This document outlined how to formulate (or strengthen), implement, evaluate compliance and assess the effectiveness of healthy public food procurement and service policies. It can be used by relevant government decision-makers or program managers at the national or regional, provincial, and municipal levels.

On February 10th, United Nations International Children's Emergency Fund (UNICEF) released the *Programme Guidance on the Prevention of Overweight and Obesity in Children and Adolescents*. This document provided strategic guidance to countries on how to adjust programming and national support to cope with changing malnutrition, including focusing on regulatory actions to improve children's food environment.

On February 25th, the *Scientific Research Report on Dietary Guidelines of Residents in China (2021)* was officially released. This report analyzed the current situation and problems of diet and nutrition health for residents in China, new evidence of diet and health research, dietary factors related to the risk reduction of main health outcomes, and key recommendations of dietary guidelines from all over the world, to promote the reasonable diet for residents in China.

On April 26th, the Dialogue on National Food Security and Sustainable Development sponsored by the Ministry of Agriculture and Rural Affairs and hosted by the China Academy of Agricultural Sciences was held in Beijing. In response to the call of the United Nations Food Systems Summit (UNFSS), with the theme of "promoting sustainable development and ensuring national food security", this conference convened a dialogue among all stakeholders in the food system at the national level. Special reports and open discussions were made on five topics, including food system transformation and policy support, food production and sustainable development, food waste reduction and impact response, food security and fair livelihood of urban and rural residents, and sustainable food consumption, to deeply explore the food security and agricultural sustainable development path in China.

On May 4th, the Food and Agriculture Organization of the United Nations (FAO) released *The 2022 Global Report on Food Crises (GRFC 2022)*. According to the report, about 193 million people in 53 countries or regions experienced food crises. The food insecurity issue was experienced by nearly 40 million people more than 2020, reaching a record high. The main causes of food insecurity were conflicts, extreme weather, and economic crisis.

On May 6th, the *White Paper on Precision Nutrition-Trends of Precision Nutrition Research and Industrial Transformation* was released. This white paper systematically summarized the frontier and application of precision nutrition research at home and abroad, deeply analyzed the opportunities and challenges faced by future research and industry, focused on the integration of Industry-University-Research, provided the industrial transformation ideas of precision nutrition solutions, and helped to build a dynamic industrial ecology.

On May 11th, the *White Paper on Healthy Cereals* was released. This white paper systematically analyzed and elucidated the consumption ways and status of healthy cereals, aiming at guiding consumers to optimize the consumption structure of cereals, increase the intake of whole grains, and help achieve the sustainable development goal of "Healthy China 2030".

On May 15th, National Nutrition Week and "5·20" China Student Nutrition Day were started in Beijing. The activity focused on the "Balanced/reasonable diet", aimed at advocating nutritious recipes, enhancing the construction of healthy families, promoting the formation and consolidation of residents' healthy diets, putting reasonable dietary action of "Health China" into practice, and forming a lifestyle of "Nutrition, Health, and No-waste" in the whole society.

On May 18th, the National Food and Nutrition Advisory Committee held the annual working meeting, which focused on the new outline, discussing new developments, constructing a new pattern, and helping to boost the improvement of food nutrition after the COVID-19 epidemic. The Institute of Food and Nutrition Development of the Ministry of Agriculture and Rural Affairs, organized experts to demonstrate the new edition of *China Food and Nutrition Development Program (2021–2035)* (draft for review). The new edition of *China Food and Nutrition Development Program (2021–2035)* will be a programmatic guiding role in promoting China's agricultural food production, transforming and upgrading the dietary structure of urban and rural residents, and building a "Healthy China" in an all-around way.

On May 31st, *White Paper on Dietary Health of White-Collar Women in China 2021* was released. This white paper mainly analyzed the food and nutrient intake and dietary structure of urban women aged 18–49 years old in China. It aims to find out the existing dietary and nutritional problems, and propose specific improvement strategies and suggestions to promote their nutrition and health.

From June 20th to August 20th, the China Youth Food System Dialogue Consultation Meeting jointly sponsored by the Institute of Food and Nutrition Development of the Ministry of Agriculture and Rural Affairs and UNICEF, was held in Chengdu and other five cities. A youth dialogue was held on the current situation and development of the food system in China. This dialogue was one of the series of activities in China in response to the UN Food System Summit. This dialogue conveyed to the world the opinions and voices of young people in China on the future food system construction, and contributed the wisdom and strength of young people in China for building a healthier, more inclusive and more sustainable food system in the future.

On July 21st, the report *Current Situation and Countermeasures of Food Nutrition Development of Children and Adolescents in China* was released. This report analyzed the current situation of children and adolescents' food nutrition development in China from three aspects: nutritional status, dietary nutrition intake and food consumption. It also puts forward seven countermeasures and suggestions, such as optimizing the dietary structure and popularizing nutrition-fortified agricultural products, which were of great significance to promote the nutritional improvement and healthy development of children and adolescents in China.

From September 9th to 11st, International Conference on Food Loss Reduction was held in Jinan. During this period, the *Jinan Initiative for International Food Loss Reduction* was released, which sent the voice of China to the world for achieving the goals of food loss reduction and food security. As a common proposition of all mankind, food security was an important guarantee for world peace and sustainable development.

On September 23rd, the first UNFSS was successfully held. The conference utilized the interrelation between the food system and global challenges such as malnutrition, climate change, poverty, etc., for promoting the progress of 17 sustainable development goals. It aimed to enable all people to make use of the power of the food system to recover from the COVID-19 epidemic, and to get life back on track. At the summit, 165 member states spoke, expounding the importance of the food system to promote the 2030 agenda at the national and global levels, calling for international and regional cooperation and economic recovery impacted by COVID-19, and ensuring the fulfillment of the promises of food security, hunger eradication, and nutrition improvement. All participants in the food system have made bold commitments, including some governments and other partners, who have made major financial commitments to support domestic and international food system reform actions, and more specific initiatives on improving nutrition and eliminating hunger. With the commitment of many parties, some multi-stakeholder initiatives and alliances have emerged to support the implementation of national and regional food system transformation, including multi-stakeholder announcements focusing on Zero hunger, Healthy eating, School feeding, Food waste reduction, and other aspects.

On September 25th, "Scaling Up Nutrition Movement (SUN) 3.0" was officially launched in Central and South Asia. SUN has covered 65 countries and 4 Indian states, which has made great progress in national nutrition. At the same time, it has played a key role in promoting the progress of global nutrition goals. As part of the United Nations Food System Summit, 53 member countries held dialogues, aimed at accelerating the construction of food systems. In addition, 60 member countries participated in the Tokyo Nutrition Promotion Growth Summit, and submitted specific and measurable commitments to the nutrition accountability framework. The year 2021 was one significant "transition and progress" of SUN. SUN 3.0 (2021－2025) has launched, indicating the beginning of the third phase of the initiative, and the opening activities were held in many member countries. At the same time, the secretariat of the

SUN was reorganized to meet the continuous development and progress needs of its members. A resource mobilization team, a strategic consulting team, and a financing capacity development platform have been set up.

On October 21st, FAO, the International Fund for Agricultural Development (IFAD), and the World Food Program (WFP) jointly implemented the *Joint Programme on Gender Transformative Approaches for Food Security and Nutrition* (*JP GTA*) through the financial support of the European Union. It proposed to achieve sustainable agriculture by addressing the root cause of gender issues. It aims to improve nutrition and food security by empowering women and realizing gender equality during transformation.

From October 30th to 31st, FAO issued the *Matera Declaration on Food Security, Nutrition, and Food System* at the G20 Summit, calling on the international community to jointly build an inclusive and resilient food system to ensure that all people get adequate nutrition, and help African countries achieve the goal of "Zero hunger" at an early date.

From October 31st to November 13th, the UK hosted the 26th United Nations Conference of the Parties to Climate Change (COP 26) in Glasgow. Nearly 200 countries gathered in the UK, pledged to take action on climate change, formulated the *Glasgow Climate Convention* to maintain the vitality of 1.5℃, and finally completed the unfinished contents of the *Paris Agreement*. The United Nations Nutrition Program Agency will work with some actors to emphasize the key role of food and nutrition in mitigating climate change, and the need to include nutrition in climate negotiations.

On November 23rd, global experts on nutrition jointly wrote and published the *Global Nutrition Report 2021*. The impact of an unhealthy diet on health and the global environment was evaluated. The financing prospect of the nutrition field was evaluated, and the progress of nutrition commitment was summarized. The report found that, although some progress was made in the global nutrition situation, the diet was not getting healthier, the requirements for the environment were getting increasingly higher, and an unacceptable level of malnutrition still existed. It was suggested that actions should be taken in three key areas: financial investment, diet and malnutrition, and accountability.

From December 7th to 8th, Tokyo Nutrition for Growth Summit was held. The summit was held in the middle of the United Nations Decade of Action on Nutrition, and there are only five years left to achieve the World Health Assembly's goals on maternal, infant and children nutrition, and ten years left to achieve the sustainable development goals. This summit identified three core fields: making nutrition an integral part of universal health insurance, establishing a food system that promoted healthy diet and nutrition, ensuring producers' livelihood and climate intelligence, and addressing malnutrition in fragile and conflict-affected situations. In addition, new common goals have been formed in these core fields, including promoting data-driven accountability and ensuring nutrition financing innovation, to support the United Nations Decade of Action on Nutrition and the sustainable development goals.

On December 29th, *Chinese Nutrition Society Expert Consensus on Dietary Fiber* was officially released. The released consensus can provide basic information for *Dietary Reference Intakes of Chinese Residents* and relevant regulations on dietary fiber, and scientifically guide food enterprises to understand and apply dietary fiber.